W9-AAL-995

DEVELOPMENTAL SPEECH AND LANGUAGE DISORDERS

THE GUILFORD CHILD PSYCHOPATHOLOGY SERIES
Thomas P. Ollendick, Editor

DEVELOPMENTAL SPEECH AND LANGUAGE DISORDERS
Dennis P. Cantwell and Lorian Baker

In preparation
EATING DISORDERS IN ADOLESCENCE
L. K. George Hsu

DEVELOPMENTAL SPEECH AND LANGUAGE DISORDERS

Dennis P. Cantwell, MD
Lorian Baker, PhD

Foreword by George Tarjan, MD

THE GUILFORD PRESS
New York London

Dedicated to

Marshall Buck, PhD

and

Susan, Suzi, Denny, Colleen, Erin, and Marianne

A Division of Guilford Publications, Inc.
200 Park Avenue South, New York, N.Y. 10003

Printed in the United States of America

10 9 8 7 6 5 4 3 2 1

Library of Congress Cataloging-in-Publication Data

Cantwell, Dennis P., 1940–
Developmental speech and language disorders.

(The Guilford child psychopathology series)
Bibliography: p.
Includes index.
1. Language disorders in children. 2. Speech disorders in children. 3. Learning disabilities. 4. Child psychopathology. I. Baker, Lorian. II. Title. III. Series. [DNLM: 1. Language Development Disorders. 2. Speech Disorders—in infancy & childhood. WM 475 C234d]
RJ496.L35C36 1987 618.92′855 86-26989
ISBN 0-89862-400-2

FOREWORD

Being a foreign medical graduate, born, reared, and educated in Hungary, coming to the United States with no practical knowledge of English impressed upon me the consequences of linguistic deficit. Gaps in linguistic knowledge can give the appearance of ignorance, rudeness, bizarreness, impoverished background, or lack of awareness. More seriously, deficits in a child's linguistic system can give the appearance of mental retardation, oppositional disorder, elective mutism, pervasive developmental disorder, environmental deprivation, or attention deficit. Yet, although linguistic functioning is considered when making a psychiatric diagnosis, it is not a major focus of psychiatric training. This book is an important step toward helping to correct this lack of emphasis.

The global nature and severity of the difficulties faced by language-impaired children is evidenced by the variety of professionals who treat them: speech/language pathologists, psychologists, reading and learning specialists, linguists, primary care physicians, neurologists, child psychiatrists, and other mental health professionals. The interdisciplinary participation of many professionals should facilitate the treatment of these children. Unfortunately, in my observation, this does not always occur. The disciplines concerned with language-impaired children are essentially isolated by disparate theoretical constructs, nosology, and methods of diagnosis and treatment. Thus, ironically, rather than cooperating to help a child, professionals from different disciplines may be driven apart by the lack of a common professional language.

Therefore, I feel that a major contribution of this book is that it gives clinicians of all backgrounds a framework for interdisciplinary integration. Further, although it is written predominantly for clinicians, it incorporates information from several different specialties, viewing the nature, assessment, and remediation of language deficits in light of the educational, emotional, and linguistic status of the child. There is a serious effort to use terminology that can accommodate the fields of speech/language pathology, psychology, psychiatry, other areas of medicine, and education.

The speech/language pathologist or educational therapist will find the DSM-III explained in such a way that the significance of the various diagnostic categories is apparent. The child psychiatrist or neurologist will find the speech and language tests summarized in such a way that the significance of good or poor performance can be determined. The child psychiatrist or pediatrician can see how the speech/language pathologist or educational psychologist does his or her assessment by asking specific questions about the child's functioning in language-related areas. In contrast, the speech/language pathologist or educational psychologist can see how the child psychiatrist makes his or her diagnosis by asking specific questions about the child's nonlinguistic functioning.

This book provides the reader with a review of the methods for assessment of the various functions of language, and a diagnosis of childhood language syndromes. Although clinically oriented, the focus of the book is not so much how to assess, diagnose, and treat language-impaired children, but rather how to approach observation, selection of assessment procedures, interpretation of assessment results, differential diagnosis, and establishment of treatment goals. By providing guidelines for decision-making, the authors in effect are teaching clinicians to think their way through diagnosis.

I read this book with great personal and professional interest. In my judgment, it will allow us to go beyond the current situation in which professionals from different backgrounds tackle isolated aspects of language deficiency to a situation in which professionals combine resources to better help language-impaired children.

George Tarjan, M.D.

PREFACE

This volume represents one product of a decade of fruitful collaboration between a psycholinguist and a child psychiatrist. At first glance, this might seem to be an unusual collaboration. Why should a psycholinguist be interested in children with psychiatric problems? Why should a child psychiatrist be interested in children with communication disorders? First, it's the ability to communicate with others that makes us uniquely human. Second, speech and language development is uniquely related to other areas of development, including cognitive development, play, learning, peer relationships, and other aspects of social and emotional development. Third, children with various types of developmental speech and language disorders make up a sizable proportion of children in the general population. And finally, children with speech and language disorders seem to be at risk for the development of both learning disorders and psychiatric disorders.

We hope that the contents of this volume are found useful by various professionals dealing with children who have communication problems. We are indebted to the many children with communication disorders and their families who have taught us much about the interrelationships of developmental speech and language disorders, developmental learning disorders, and psychiatric disorders. We are also indebted to Seymour Weingarten of Guilford Press for his enthusiastic acceptance of the idea of this volume.

The preparation of this volume was aided by funds from the Catherine Davis Trust and by Grants Nos. 17371 and 35116 from the National Institute of Mental Health.

A word on pronoun usage in the volume is in order here. We use the pronouns "he," "his," and so on to refer to "a child" or "a person" in the generic sense. No sexism is intended; the masculine form is used purely as a less awkward alternative to "he and she" and the like.

Finally, we wish to note that the order of authorship of this volume is arbitrary and does not reflect our differential contributions to the work.

Dennis P. Cantwell
Lorian Baker

CONTENTS

CHAPTER 1

Introduction, Definitions, and Epidemiology

Introduction

This volume is written for professionals, and in particular for clinicians, who work with children with delayed or disordered speech or language development. Since such professionals come from diverse backgrounds, we have tried to limit the terminology and theoretical discussions to those necessary for an understanding of the basic clinical issues.

The volume is divided into seven chapters. Chapter 1 provides a brief discussion of the definitions, classifications, and epidemiology of the developmental speech and language disorders. The appendix to Chapter 1 is a list of definitions used throughout the book. Chapter 2 outlines the pattern of acquisition of speech and language in the normal child. Chapter 3 discusses methods of assessment, both formal and informal, that are used in establishing the diagnoses of developmental language or articulation disorders. Chapter 4 provides clinical descriptions of various syndromes involving abnormal language or speech development, and gives guidelines for making differential diagnoses according to criteria of the third edition of the *Diagnostic and Statistical Manual of Mental Disorders* (DSM-III) (American Psychiatric Association, 1980). Chapter 5 provides some case illustrations of children with syndromes involving abnormal or delayed speech or language development, and discussion of the cases in terms of diagnosis and treatment plans. Chapter 6 summarizes what is known about the effects of developmental articulation and language disorders on the psychiatric and educational status of the child. Finally, Chapter 7 suggests possible treatment and intervention strategies.

Overview of Definitions and Etiological Hypotheses

"Developmental language disorder" is a disturbance or delay in language acquisition that is unexplained by general mental retardation, hearing impairment, neurological impairments, or physical abnormalities. "Developmental articulation disorder" is the frequent and recurrent misarticulation of speech sounds resulting in speech that is considered abnormal when compared to that of peers.

Despite the early identification of developmental language disorder (the first references were made in the early 1800s) and the continuing involvement of professionals from a variety of disciplines, the nature and definition of the disorder are still unclear. The first groups of professionals interested in specific childhood language disorders were neurologists and aphasiologists. Their work centered on comparing the language disorders found in children to those found in adult patients who had sustained brain injuries (Gall, 1825; Vaisse, 1866). The view that similar mechanisms (in particular, lesions in similar areas of the brain) must be involved in childhood and adult language impairments was reflected in the use of terms such as "infantile aphasia" and "congenital aphasia." Ongoing attempts to establish and/or localize abnormal brain functioning in children with developmental language disorder have included examinations of electroencephalographic (EEG) tracings (Maccario, Hefferen, Keblusek, & Lipinski, 1982; Sato & Dreifuss, 1973), cerebral autopsies (Goldstein, 1974; Landau, Goldstein, & Kleffner, 1960), and dominance or lateralization (Annett, 1981; Kinsbourne, 1979; Witelson & Rabinovitz, 1972; Zaidel, 1979).

Through the mid-1900s, the view of the childhood language disorder changed from a neurological to a developmental focus. It was recognized that, rather than *losing* language, these children actually suffer from a failure to *develop* language normally. Concurrent with this shift in focus was the introduction of descriptive developmental terms such as "dysphasia," "developmental childhood aphasia," "minimal brain damage," and "oligophasia." The assumption of most authors using these terms was that diffuse, unlocalized, or subclinical neurological dysfunctions, if not overt lesions, were responsible for the disordered language. The prevalence of abnormal neurological "soft signs," including motor coordination problems and attentional problems in children with developmental language disorder, has been cited in support of this hypothesis.

In the mid-1900s, a psycholinguistic approach to developmental language disorders occurred. Psychologists, focusing on the perceptual functioning of these children, introduced terms such as "congenital auditory imperception," "congenital word deafness," "developmental word deafness," and "congenital verbal auditory agnosia" as descriptors. Linguists, focusing on descriptions of the actual disordered behavior involved, used terms such as "developmental language disorder," "language disability," "delayed language," "language retardation," "linguistic delay," "linguistic retardation," "delayed language development," and "deviant language."

The approach of the perceptual psychologists supposes that the underlying difficulties in developmental language disorder are not problems with language concepts or grammatical rules per se, but rather problems involving such basic skills as perception, discrimination, memory, or association. The auditory–perceptual deficits that have been posited as underlying include defects in auditory attention span (Aram & Nation, 1982; Semel, 1976); sorting out "background" versus "significant" auditory signals (Costello, 1977; Keir, 1977; Lasky & Tobin, 1973); discriminating speech sounds, acoustic signals, or speech sounds in context (Eisenson, 1968; Mark & Hardy, 1958; McReynolds, 1967; Semel, 1976); discriminating speech sounds at the rate at which they normally occur (Frumkin & Rapin, 1979; Tallal, 1978); storing speech sounds, sound contexts, or words (Eisenson, 1968; Keir, 1977; Masland & Case, 1968; Rosenthal, 1972; Wiig & Semel, 1980); processing sequenced materials (Eisenson, 1966; Lowe & Campbell, 1965; Monsees, 1961, 1968); scanning and associating auditory and visual stimuli (Chapanis, 1977); and discriminating rhythmic material (P. Griffiths, 1972; Kracke, 1975). The linguistic hypotheses have derived from grammatical analyses of the language of children with developmental language disorder, which suggest that these children suffer from deficits specific to the handling of certain linguistic units (Eisenson & Ingram, 1972; Johnston & Kahmi, 1980; Lee, 1974; Leonard, 1972; Menyuk, 1964; Morehead & Ingram, 1973; Wiig & Semel, 1976a, 1980).

As with developmental language disorder, there have also been a variety of terms to describe developmental articulation disorder, and a variety of hypotheses as to etiology. These terms include "baby talk," "lalling," "dyslalia," "functional speech disorder," "specific developmental speech disorder," "infantile articulation," "lazy speech," "oral inaccuracy," and "phonological impairment." The factors that have been postulated as playing a role in the etiology of the disorder (Winitz, 1969) include cognitive deficits; deficits in auditory–perceptual abilities; deficits in general motor skills or oral motor skills; speech mechanism abnormalities; social or environmental limitations; and general developmental lags.

Overview of DSM-III and Other Classification Systems

There has also been a lack of consensus on the definitions and classification systems for childhood speech and language disorders. In the present work, the DSM-III (American Psychiatric Association, 1980) framework for classification is used. DSM-III is a categorical (rather than a dimensional) system of classification, which uses an atheoretical, phenomenological descriptive approach. In DSM-III, disorders are systematically described in terms of essential features, associated features, age of onset, course, impairment, complications, predisposing factors, prevalence, sex ratio, familial pattern, and differential diagnosis. This description is followed by specific diagnostic criteria that spell out the essential features for the diagnosis of each disorder. There is no attempt to account for the etiology of disorders.

Each of the disorders in DSM-III is conceptualized as a clinically significant behavioral or psychological syndrome—that is, a pattern that occurs in an individual and that is typically associated with either a painful symptom (distress) or an impairment (disability) in some important area of functioning. For each of the disorders in DSM-III, there is the inference of a behavioral, psychological, or biological dysfunction; in other words, it is inferred that the disturbance is not solely in the relationship between the individual and society.

The term "syndrome" is used in a somewhat unusual way in DSM-III. In this use of the term, there is no requirement of postdictive validity (i.e., that the symptoms can be shown to be the result of a specific etiological influence) or concurrent validity (i.e., that the syndrome can be differentiated in ways other than the core symptoms—e.g., by natural history, family pattern of psychopathology, or association with other disorders). Nor is there any requirement for a unitary cluster of characteristics, a common cause, or a consistent response to treatment, which have been suggested by several authors (Ross & Ross, 1982; Shaffer & Greenhill, 1979) as requirements for syndrome status. The syndromes described in DSM-III have face validity, descriptive validity, and predictive validity, permitting one to make a prediction about the natural history of the disorder.

In this sense, the developmental speech and language disorders are classified on Axis II of a five-axis scheme, under the heading "specific developmental disorders." The other specific developmental disorders of DSM-III include developmental reading disorder, developmental arithmetic disorder, "mixed" specific developmental disorder, and "atypical" developmental disorder. These developmental disorders are viewed as disorders of specific areas of development that are not due to another mental disorder. Although it is recognized that each area of development is related to biological maturation, there is no assumption regarding the primacy of biological etiological factors, and nonbiological factors are presumed to be involved in many, if not all, of these disorders.

The inclusion of the category of "specific developmental disorders" in an overall classification of "mental disorders" has been controversial. Indeed, many children with these specific developmental disorders have no other signs of clinical psychopathology, and detection and treatment usually do not take place in a psychiatric setting. Nevertheless, these conditions are classified in the "mental disorder" section of the ninth edition of the *International Classification of Diseases* (ICD-9) (World Health Organization, 1977), and they do fall within the broad DSM-III concept of "mental disorder" as described above—that is, a clinically significant behavioral or psychological syndrome, causing some degree of distress, disability, and disadvantage.

Currently DSM-III is under review, and a revised version is planned for publication sometime in 1987. In the revised version of DSM-III (DSM-IIIR), the coding of Axis II will be changed, and the name of the axis will be "developmental disorders" rather than "specific developmental disorders." The following disorders will be included as developmental disorders in DSM-IIIR: mental retardation, pervasive developmental disorders, specific developmental disorders (which will include language and speech disorders, academic skills disorders, and motor skills disorders, and "other developmental disorders."

In DSM-III (and in the present work), a distinction is maintained between "speech" (the physical process by which sounds are uttered) and "language" (the more complex system of arbitrary symbols that acts as a code for representing messages). Language is viewed as involving a number of subsystems: words and their associated meanings; rules for combining words into sentences; and rules for using sentences in discourse. Developmental articulation disorder is conceptualized as a disruption involving speech acquisition, whereas developmental language disorder is viewed as a disruption involving primarily some aspect of language acquisition.

Other classification systems for syndromes involving childhood speech and language development have included those of Adler (1964), Aram and Nation (1982), Chase (1972), Culbertson, Norlin, and Ferry (1981), Ingram (1972),

McGrady (1968), Morley (1957), Myklebust (1954), Orton (1937), Perkins (1977), Pirozzolo, Campanella, Christensen, and Lawson-Kerr (1981), and Wood (1964). Such models have ranged from the purely descriptive (which classify disorders according to the areas of development they affect—e.g., reading, word deafness, or motor speech) to the etiological (which classify disorders according to their presumed cause—e.g., mental retardation, hearing loss, or neurological deficits). One interesting and, we feel, very promising approach to this problem of classification is that of Martin (1980), who concludes that, at the present time, any classification systems are premature. Martin suggests the collection of further data prior to the delineation of specific syndromes, using formulas that rate, on a 3-point (normal to severely abnormal) scale, speech (voice, fluency, articulation), verbal expression, hearing, verbal comprehension, and nonverbal comprehension. We feel that such an approach would prove useful not only for classifying all childhood communication disorders, but for describing subtypes of developmental language disorder as well.

Currently, most authors recognize that developmental language disorder is not a single entity, but a collective term for a range of abnormal development involving differing aspects of speech and language. The earliest approach (Morley, 1957; Pirozzolo *et al.*, 1981), and the one that DSM-III follows, is that there are two major subtypes of the disorder: an "expressive" subtype (which is less severe, involving an impairment in the encoding or production of language, while the understanding of language remains intact) and a "receptive" subtype (which is more severe, involving impairment of the understanding of language). Other classification schemes accepting the "receptive" versus "expressive" distinction but attaching additional subtypes include those of Myklebust (1954), Strauss (1954), McGinnis, Kleffner, and Goldstein (1956), and Ingram (1972). More recent approaches have ignored subclassifications based upon either the "receptive" versus "expressive" or the severity distinctions, and have attempted, using linguistic terms, to delineate the areas of language that are affected (Bloom & Lahey, 1978; Tomblin, 1978; Wiig & Semel, 1980).

Epidemiology

Partially because of the difficulties with the definitions of speech and language disorders, the prevalence of both developmental language disorder and developmental articulation disorder is unclear. The literature shows a wide range in prevalence estimates: from a low of 0.2% to a high of 13% for developmental language disorder, and from a low of 1% to a high of 21% for developmental articulation disorder. A conservative estimate is that approximately 10% of children aged 3–7 years have developmental articulation disorder and that approximately 5% of children aged 8 years and above have developmental language disorder.

Despite the fact that there is considerable disagreement on prevalence figures for developmental speech and language disorders, there is surprising agreement across studies regarding certain etiological data. For example, it is known that there is a regular and marked decrease in the frequency of developmental articulation disorder as children increase in age. It is also known that developmental articulation disorder is more common in boys than girls, with two to three boys being affected for every one girl.

The distribution of developmental language disorder shows approximately three males being affected for every female. While family histories of developmental language disorder in first-degree relatives are not common, there is evidence that the child with a positive family history for any developmental disorders, especially developmental reading disorder or developmental articulation disorder, is more at risk for developmental language disorder than is the child with a negative family history. Several authors have also reported that children with developmental language disorder have a disproportionate amount of left-handedness or ambidexterity in their family histories.

Appendix A. Definitions

Affricate: A speech sound composed of a stop sound and a fricative sound. Examples are /ch/ as in "chew," (which is composed of /t/ and /sh/ sounds) and /dg/ as in "judge."

Ambiguous: Words or utterances whose meaning can be understood in more than one way.

Anomia: Partial loss of the ability to name objects or to recall and recognize names (or nouns). Also called "dysnomia."

Aphasia: Disorder involving loss of some or all language skills as a result of acquired brain damage. (Used by some authors to refer to "developmental language disorder.")

Apraxia: Inability to execute voluntary motor acts. Usually refers to oral apraxia, or the inability to execute speech sounds.

Articulation: Movement and placement during speech of the lips, tongue, jaw, epiglottis, and/or vocal cords in order to form speech sounds.

Astereognosis: Inability to determine the shape of an object through feeling. Usually refers to oral astereognosis, which is tested by placement of different-shaped objects in the mouth.

Attention: Ability to focus in a sustained manner on a particular task or activity for a long time. When attention is drawn frequently to unimportant or to irrelevant stimuli, an individual may be characterized as being easily distractible. Sustained attention and distractibility are interrelated but distinct abilities.

Audiology: Study of hearing, concerned with the nature of hearing, the identification of hearing loss, the assessment of hearing loss, and the rehabilitation of hearing impairment.

Auditory discrimination: Ability to recognize and distinguish the similarities and differences between sounds (usually speech sounds, or phonemes).

Auditory figure–ground: Ability to distinguish relevant auditory messages from competing irrelevant or background messages.

Auditory memory: Ability to store and retrieve heard information.

Auditory memory span: Number of related items (usually words or digits) that can be recalled immediately after hearing them presented.

Auditory perception: Mental awareness of sound; sometimes used as synonymous with "auditory discrimination."

Auditory processing: Act of receiving, perceiving, and interpreting spoken language. Types of auditory processing skills are auditory attention, auditory discrimination, and auditory memory.

Auditory sequencing: Ability to recognize the order in which sounds are heard.

Autism: Disorder characterized by three major symptoms: pervasive lack of responsiveness to other people, serious deficits in language development, and ritualistic compulsive behavior. Also used to refer to the symptom of pervasive lack of responsiveness to other people.

Babbling: Stage in the acquisition of speech during which the infant engages in a kind of vocal play involving the repetitive production of speech sounds with intonation patterns of sentences.

Bilabial: Consonant sound formed with the aid of both lips. Examples are /p/, /b/, and /m/.

Blocking: A psychiatric term referring to pauses in speech occurring before a thought or idea has been completed. Typically, after blocking, the speaker will say either spontaneously or upon questioning that he cannot recall what he has been saying.

Ceiling: Level on a standardized test at which the test becomes insensitive to further changes in performance.

Circumstantiality: A psychiatric term for speech that is indirect and delayed in reaching the point because of many unnecessary and meticulous details, although the speaker maintains his awareness of the original topic.

Clanging: A pattern of speech in which word choices are governed by sounds rather than by conceptual relationships. The speech may include rhymes and puns.

Cluttering: A disorder of speech fluency involving both the rate and rhythm of speech, and resulting in impaired speech intelligibility. Speech is erratic and dysrhythmic, consisting of rapid and jerky spurts that usually involve faulty phrasing patterns.

Cognition: Process of structuring and synthesizing the characteristics of perceived data.

Comprehension: Understanding of the semantic or syntactic aspects of language. Same as "language comprehension" and "receptive language."

Communication: Exchange of ideas, intentions, or information by means of verbal or nonverbal actions. A broader and more inclusive term than "language" or "speech."

Communicative intent: Desire to convey meanings to others.

Consonant: Speech sound produced by contractions of the articulatory muscles that modify, interrupt, or obstruct the expired air stream to the extent that its pressure is raised.

Decibel (dB): Unit of sound intensity. Named after Alexander Graham Bell. The decibel is equal to approximately one "just-noticeable" difference of loudness.

Delayed speech: Delays in speech or language milestones, particularly age of first word. Sometimes used as a synonym for "developmental language disorder."

Delusion: A fixed false belief based on an incorrect inference about external reality, which is held by an individual despite the presence of obvious proof or evidence to the contrary. To be considered a delusion, the belief must not be one that is ordinarily accepted by members of the individual's subculture, such as members of a religious group. Delusions are generally classified according to their content, and can be considered as disorders of thought content as opposed to formal thought disorders.

Denasality: Vocal quality when the nasal passages are obstructed to prevent adequate nasal resonance during speech. For example, "a code in de dose" ("a cold in the nose").

Dental: Speech sounds made by tongue (or lip) contact with the teeth. For example, /d/, /n/, and /t/ are "pure" dental sounds; /f/ and /v/ are labiodental sounds.

Developmental articulation disorder: Frequent and recurrent misarticulation of speech sounds, resulting in speech that is considered abnormal when compared to the speech of other children of the same age and from the same linguistic community. Historically, the following terms are synonymous: "baby talk," "lalling," "dyslalia," "functional articulation disorder," "specific developmental speech disorder," "infantile articulation," and "lazy speech."

Developmental language disorder: Disturbance or delay in the acquisition of language that cannot be explained by general mental retardation, hearing impairment, neurological impairments, or physical abnormalities. Historically, the following terms are synonymous: "dysphasia," "developmental childhood aphasia," "minimal brain damage," "oligophasia," "congenital auditory imperception," "developmental word deafness," "language retardation," "delayed language development," and "language disability."

Developmental language disorder, expressive subtype: Subtype of developmental language disorder in which understanding of language is normal, but expressive skills, such as the production of words and sentences, are impaired. Sometimes called "expressive dysphasia."

Developmental language disorder, receptive subtype: Subtype of developmental language disorder in which the understanding of language is impaired. Sometimes called "receptive dysphasia."

Diadochokinesis: Ability to start and alternatively stop the rapid movement of the articulators, as is required in rapidly repeating syllables such as "tut-tut-tut" or "puh-tuh-kuh."

Dysarthria: Impairment of speech articulation caused by organic abnormalities involving the speech mechanism.

Dysfluency: Any disruptions in the flow of speech involving repetitions or prolongations of words or sounds; hesitations or pauses within or between utterances; or, specifically, the "normal stuttering" found in the early speech of some children who are generally unaware of their lack of fluency.

Dyslalia: Early term for developmental articulation disorder.

Dyslexia: Disorder of reading resulting in reading skills significantly below the levels predicted by intellectual capacity and not the result of inadequate schooling. Referred to in DSM-III as "developmental reading disorder."

Dysphasia: Term currently used throughout Great Britain, and sometimes in the United States, as a synonym for "developmental language disorder."

Echolalia: Repetition or "echoing" of words or phrases previously heard. Usually refers to immediate echolalia, or the repeating of words or phrases that have just been heard. May refer to delayed echolalia, or the repetition of utterances heard some time in the past.

Egocentric speech: Self-directed speech normally found in children during the early stages of language acquisition.

Elective mutism: Disorder defined in DSM-III as the continuous refusal to talk in almost all social situations, including at school, with the ability to comprehend spoken language and to speak, and not due to another mental or physical disorder. Also sometimes called "selective mutism."

Expression: Process of formulating ideas into words and sentences in accordance with the set of grammatical and semantic rules of the language. Also sometimes called "language production."

Figure–ground: See "auditory figure–ground."

Flight of ideas: A psychiatric term for rapid speech in a nearly continuous flow, which includes abrupt topic changes usually based on understandable associations, word plays, or distracting stimuli. Severe flight of ideas may lead to a disorganized and incoherent pattern of speech.

Fricative: Speech sound produced by forcing an air stream through a narrow opening and resulting in audible high-frequency vibrations. Examples are /f/, /th/, and /v/.

Grammar: Rules by which morphemes can be strung into words and words can be strung together into sentences.

Graphemes: Written forms (or "letters") that represent speech sounds, or "phonemes."

Hallucination: A sensory perception that occurs in the absence of external stimulation of the relevant sensory organ. May be auditory, gustatory, olfactory, somatic, tactile, or visual. Hallucinations generally do not refer to the type of false perceptions that occur during dreaming or while awakening or falling asleep, and are distinguished from illusions, in which there is an external stimulus, but that external stimulus is misperceived or misinterpreted.

Hertz (Hz): Unit of the frequency of sounds equal to one cycle per second.

High-frequency hearing loss: Hearing impairment involving only the high-frequency sounds.

Holophrastic speech: One- or two-word utterances of children in the early stages of language acquisition, which are believed to express more complex meanings.

Hypernasality: Speech characterized by excessive nasal resonance. Occurs frequently in cases of cleft palate.

Idiom: Phrase or expression whose meaning contrasts with the meaning of the individual words.

Illogical thinking: Psychiatric term referring to thinking in which conclusions are reached that are clearly false, given initial premises, and that contain clear internal contradictions. Illogical thinking may be observed in the absence or the presence of delusional thinking.

Incoherent speech: Psychiatric term referring to speech that is not understandable because of one or more of the following situations: lack of logical connection between words, phrases, and sentences; excessive use of incomplete sentences; distorted grammar; abrupt changes in subject matter; or idiosyncratic usage of words. Incoherent speech is not considered to be present when the disturbance is purely due to aphasia.

Infantile autism: See "autism."

Inner language: Acquisition of concepts, as distinct from the acquisition of verbal labels for such concepts. The presence of inner language in a young child may be inferred by meaningful use of objects and presence of pretend play.

Intonation: Pitch contours and stress patterns of utterances. In English, an intonation pattern involving falling pitch at the end of an utterance usually marks a statement, and an intonation pattern involving rising pitch at the end of an utterance marks a question. Intonation patterns may also convey uncertainty, resignation, disapproval, or boredom.

Jargon: Use of strings of sounds or "made-up words" that apparently have meaning to the young child acquiring language.

Labial: Speech sounds produced with the aid of the lips. Includes bilabial sounds (/p/, /b/, and /m/) and labiodental (/f/, /v/) sounds.

Language: System of arbitrary symbols (vocal or otherwise) to represent meanings.

Language processing: Act of receiving, perceiving and interpreting language. The term is often used synonymously with "auditory processing."

Language production: See "expression."

Lexical: Having to do with the words (or vocabulary) of a language.

Linguistic concepts: Logical relationships between the words in a sentence. Examples include "if–then," "all–but," "when–then," "not–any."

Lisping: Defective production of sibilant sounds.

Loose associations: A psychiatric term for communications characterized by shifts from one subject to another that are either totally unrelated or only very obliquely related to each other, and in which the speaker does not show any awareness that the topics are unconnected to each other.

Mental retardation (DSM-III definition): Condition with onset before age 18 and characterized by general intellectual functioning that is below 70 (full-scale intelligence score on standardized test), and by concurrent impairments in adaptive functioning.

Morpheme: Smallest unit of language capable of bearing meaning. In English the morpheme frequently is a word, but often it can be part of a word. For example, the -s on the end of a word to denote the plural is a morpheme.

Nasal: Pertaining to the nose; also, a voiced speech sound with nasal resonance (e.g., /m/, /n/, and /n/).

Neologisms: Use of words in a highly idiosyncratic way, considering the educational and cultural background of the speaker.

Nouns: Words that label.

Overextension: See "overgeneralization."

Overgeneralization: Use of a word by a child to refer to a wider meaning than the correct meaning for the word. For example, the child may use the word "Rover" to refer to any dog, or the word "dog" to refer to any animal. Also called "overextension."

Perseveration: Continuing references to earlier topics or responses.

Phoneme: Basic discernible segment in the sound pattern of a language; a speech sound.

Phonetic: Having to do with the acoustic and articulatory characteristics of speech sounds.

Phonology: Study of the rules for combining and selecting the speech sounds of a language.

Pitch: Fundamental frequency of the voice during speech. Also called "tone."

Poverty of speech: A psychiatric term referring to a restriction in the amount of speech manifested by brief, unelaborated spontaneous speech and brief unelaborated replies to questions; poverty of content of speech; or speech that is not restricted in quantity but conveys little new information because of frequent use of obscure phrases, stereotyped phrases, repetitions, or vagueness. Generally, this term is not used if speech is incoherent.

Pragmatics: The way in which an individual uses language to communicate.

Pressure of speech: A psychiatric term referring to speech that is increased in amount, rapid in rate, and difficult to interpret.

Prosody: Melodic features of speech, superimposed on the ongoing stream of speech, which signal differences in meanings. The prosodic features of speech include variations in pitch and stress.

Psychosis: Disorder characterized by gross impairment in reality testing, so that an individual does not correctly evaluate the accuracy of his perceptions and thoughts, but makes incorrect inferences about external reality. The term "psychotic" may be used to describe the behavior of a particular individual at a particular point in time. The term "psychosis" is used to describe the set of mental disorders in which a gross impairment in reality testing occurs at some time during the course of the illness.

Pure tone: A sound consisting of a single frequency.

Question transformation: Derivation of a question from an active declarative sentence by changing the word order.

Receptive: Ability to comprehend or understand the meaning of words or sentences heard.

Semantics: Meanings of words and sentences.

Semantic class: Groups of words that are related in meaning.

Sibilant: A type of fricative speech sound that involves a "hissing" quality. Examples are /s/, /z/, /sh/, /ch/, and /dg/.

Sign language: System of communication used by the deaf, in which the fingers and hands are used as articulators to form signs or gestures that represent ideas, objects, attributes, or actions.

Speech: Physical (motor or articulatory) process by which the sounds of a language are uttered.

Speech pathologist: Professional with training in the evaluation and treatment of speech and language disorders. Also called "speech-language pathologist."

Stop: Speech sound produced when the air stream is blocked. Examples are /p/, /b/, /t/, /d/, /g/, and /k/.

Stress: Relatively increased loudness of some syllables as compared with others.

Stuttering: Any disruptions in the flow of speech involving repetitions or prolongations of words or sounds; hesitations or pauses within or between utterances; or, specifically, disruptions of speech when accompanied by awareness, anxiety, or compensatory behaviors.

Syntax: Organizational rules for generating and interpreting sentence structures.

Telegraphic language: Sentences found in the speech of children following the "two-word utterance" stage of language acquisition, in which words not essential for conveying meaning are omitted.

Thought disorder: A generic term for a disorder of thought content (essentially delusions) or a disorder of the form of thought (or formal thought disorder). Sometimes called "formal thought disorder." The diagnosis of thought disorder is generally made on the basis of abnormalities in speech, language, and communication, but the boundaries of the concept of formal thought disorder are not clear. It has recently been suggested that (in addition to disorders of form and content of thought), subtypes of thought disorder may include disorders of stream of thought ("blocking") and disorders of possession of thought.

Tongue-tie: Rare condition of limited movement of the tongue, due to abnormal shortness of the lingual frenum.

Tongue-thrust: Anterior thrusting of the tongue during swallowing.

Transformations: Syntactic operations involving manipulation of elements of sentences in order to derive complex sentence types such as passives, negatives, and interrogatives from "simple" active declarative sentences.

Underextension: Use of a word to refer only to some narrow subset of its "true" meaning (e.g., using the word "car" to mean only "moving cars").

Vocalizations: Nonspeech sounds produced by a person.

Vowel: Sounds produced with little obstruction to the air stream.

CHAPTER 2

Normal Development of Speech and Language

Introduction

An understanding of the stages occurring in normal speech and language development is necessary in order to recognize abnormal or delayed speech or language development.

Normative data on childhood speech and language acquisition suggest that both of these processes follow specific stages of development (Bloom, 1978; B. B. Brown, 1973; H. H. Clark & Clark, 1977; Dale, 1976; De Villiers & De Villiers, 1978). Speech articulation, for example, goes through stages in an orderly pattern, beginning with vocalization and progressing through systematic acquisition of speech sounds. Language acquisition also follows a pattern of stages, beginning with a prelinguistic stage and continuing through a single-word stage, a two-word message stage, a simplified-sentences stage, and a grammar development stage, and finally developing into varied and complex language used for a range of communicative functions.

There is some overlapping between the stages of language development; that is, the stages are not completely discontinuous steps in development marked by clear divisions. Nonetheless, these stages represent a method of conceptualizing speech and language acquisition as manageable units for discussion.

Below, a general description of the stages involved in speech and language acquisition is given, along with the major features of each stage. Readers interested in more detailed descriptions of speech and language development are referred to the following works: Bloom (1970, 1973), B. B. Brown (1973), Cromer (1980), Dale (1976), Eisenson (1972), Golinkoff (1983), Greenfield and Smith (1976), Howlin (1980), Karmiloff-Smith (1979), McNeill, (1970), Menyuk (1976), Palermo and Molfese (1972), and Reynell (1979).

Research on language acquisition shows that there is a wide range of "normal" development (Bowerman, 1978; Meline & Meline, 1981; Nelson, 1981). The precise nature of individual differences in language acquisition is now only beginning to be understood, but it appears that within the various stages of development, different items and different orders of acquisition may occur. The relationship between the acquisition of language comprehension and language expression skills is also unclear. Some researchers believe that the acquisition of skills in comprehension precedes the acquisition of skills in expression (Fraser, Bellugi, & Brown, 1963; Nelson, 1973), whereas other researchers believe the opposite (R. Chapman & Miller, 1975).

In our discussion of speech and language development below, we define the different stages of acquisition in general terms, and indicate a corresponding age range during which this acquisition generally occurs in normal children. In order to judge whether a child's speech or language acquisition is within normal limits, the clinician should look both for an appropriate age of acquisition and for consistency within a stage of development. While some variation is normal, a child should have most of the skills listed for his age level. Scattered development across several stages, and/or overall delays of more than 6 months, are causes for concern.

Development of Speech Articulation Skills

The development of speech articulation skills follows a pattern of six general stages. Even in the prelinguistic phase, before the child uses his first words to communicate, several stages of development occur. Once the child utters his first word, his sound system forms in an orderly manner.

Below, the general stages of speech articulation acquisition are summarized. Readers interested in more detailed information on the acquisition of speech articulation skills are directed to the following works: Albright and Albright (1956), Eisenson (1963), Ferguson (1978), McReynolds (1978), and Winitz (1969).

The Early Vocalization Stage (1–4 Months of Age)

In the first months of life, the only vocalizations made by the infant are cries. There is some controversy as to whether the neonate produces different cries to indicate different desires. While parents frequently report that they can recognize "happy," "angry," "hungry," or "pained" cries in their newborn infants, research has been unable to verify these claims (Muller, Hollien, & Murray, 1974).

At any rate, within a month or so after birth, the infant produces vocalizations other than crying, and the frequency of crying diminishes. Vocalizations clearly showing contentment, as opposed to distress, occur (Ricks, 1975). These early vocalizations have been called "cooing" and "gurgling" because they generally consist of vowels and consonants that are formed in the back of the mouth, such as those found in the words "coo" and "gurgle."

The Babbling and "Playing with Sounds" Stage (3–15 Months of Age)

Starting at approximately 3–4 months of age, the infant begins to produce sounds that more clearly approximate speech. A variety of consonants and vowels can be heard, and an "intonation pattern" (or rising and falling pattern of voice pitches, and stress and rhythmic changes) is imposed upon the strings of consonants and vowels. The earliest babbling consists of vowels such as those found in the words "cat" and "cup"; a full range of vowel and consonant sounds is used by the infant. Research suggests that babbling is universal and consists of the same sounds and patterns, regardless of the language to which the infant is exposed (Ferguson, 1978). Even babies who have deaf–mute parents and babies who are deaf themselves begin babbling in the same way.

The first intonation patterns used in babbling are typically rising patterns, which give the impression that the baby is attempting to converse in his own language. Later, rising and falling intonation patterns are used, as well as patterns of final stress, which produce the impression that the baby is sometimes making statements, sometimes asking questions, and sometimes demanding something "right now" (Menyuk, 1971).

As babbling becomes firmly established in the infant, a period of "playing with sounds" can be detected. The infant is able to mimic the intonation and sound patterns that his parents produce and may often be found engaging in self-imitation. Motor imitations may occur to accompany the speech imitations, so that the baby may be able to "wave bye-bye" while saying "bye." At this stage of development, babies also make eye contact with their parents and vocalize simultaneously or in alternation with the parents (Bateson, 1975; Stern, Jaffe, Beebe, & Bennett, 1975). Toward the end of this stage, the infant gives indications of recognizing his own name, and may often begin babbling when he hears his own name. Also, the baby may spend considerable amounts of time "talking to himself" in long patterns of sounds.

Observational studies suggest that infant babbling is usually accompanied by motor movements, particularly eye gazing. It has been proposed that babbling is a necessary precursor to language development (Mowrer, 1960; Oller, Wieman, Doyle, & Ross, 1976), although there are no conclusive data available to confirm this. Attempts have been made to correlate type and amount of babbling with family environment, social class, intelligence levels, and developmental factors, but there are no definitive results (H. H. Clark & Clark, 1977; Nakazima, 1975).

The First Speech Sounds (11–18 Months of Age)

Sometime around the child's first birthday, there is a decrease in the large number and combinations of speech sounds that the child produces, and at about this time, the child says his first word (Darley & Winitz, 1961). Occasionally, there may be a brief period when the child stops vocalizing altogether, although more commonly there is no clear-cut transition from babbling to "real words."

Regardless of which language a child is learning, his first words are produced from a limited set of sounds—usually a consonant produced in the front of the mouth (such as /p/, /b/, /t/, /d/, or /m/) and a vowel (Jakobson, 1968). The first words are frequently simple consonant-plus-vowel (CV) combinations, such as "ma" ("Mama"), "ba" ("bottle"), and "da" ("dog"), or repeated syllables ("reduplicated syllables," CVCV), such as "mama," "baba," or "dada."

Systematic Acquisition of Speech Sounds (18–50 Months of Age)

The child's production of sounds in "true" speech (i.e., in words with meaning) differs from his production of sounds during the babbling stage of development. First, babbling consists of a wide range of sounds, whereas speech acquisition begins with a smaller set of sounds gradually increased. Second, in babbling, an almost infinite number of sequential combinations of sounds is produced, whereas in speech acquisition, only limited combinations of sounds are produced.

In fact, the child's acquisition of speech skills is an amazingly systematic process (Ferguson, 1978). As we have stated, the first speech sounds that the child uses with meaning are "frontal" consonants such as /p/, /b/, and /m/, and vowels. Vowel sounds are mastered quickly (in the first 18 months of age), whereas the full inventory of consonant sounds is not mastered for several years. Studies have shown that for English (and possibly universally), correct production of consonant sounds occurs in a more or less systematic order.

Although there is considerable variation among normal children in the acquisition of sounds in words, there is still a general pattern of acquisition that is followed whereby certain sounds are acquired by certain ages. Several studies (Poole, 1934; Sander, 1972; Templin, 1957) have been done to determine which speech sounds are "mastered" (correctly produced by 75% of children) at various ages, and the results of such studies can provide useful guidelines of "normal" articulatory acquisition. Table 2-1 presents a summary of these guidelines.

Because the child's early speech is produced with only a limited set of speech sounds, the speech of a young child frequently sounds like a garbled version of adult speech. The interpretation services of the child's mother may be necessary in order for the nonfamily member to understand what the young child is saying. In fact, it has been estimated that only 25% of the utterances of the average 20-month-old child, and only 50% of the 30-month-old's utterances, are intelligible.

Yet, upon closer examination, it turns out that there is regularity and patterning in the child's speech. The errors found in the child's articulation of speech sounds are not random, but rather follow "rules" (De Villiers & De Villiers, 1978; Kahn, 1982). Such rules or normal errors in the articulation of the young child include the following:

1. Omitting the last consonant sound or sounds of a word (e.g., saying "ka" for "cat," "ba" for "ball").
2. "Devoicing" consonants (substituting /p/ for /b/, /t/ for /d/, /k/ for /g/, or /f/ for /v/).
3. "Stopping" consonants (substituting /b/ for /v/, /p/ for /f/, /t/ for /th/, /d/ for /th/).
4. "Gliding" consonants (substituting /w/ or /y/ for /l/ or /r/).
5. "Reducing" consonant clusters (substituting a single consonant for a group of consonants; e.g., saying "top" for "stop," "mall" for "small," "mik" for "milk," "tet" for "tent," "bu" for "blue").
6. Omitting unstressed syllables in words of two or more syllables (e.g., saying "raf" for "giraffe," "fant" for "elephant").

Not all children use all of these rules with equal frequency. There have been some suggestions that children may select "favorite" sounds or rules when acquiring speech (Ferguson, 1978).

When one is attempting to understand the speech of young children, it is helpful to keep in mind these simplifying rules, and to remember that a combination of several of these rules may be applied to each word, producing speech that may

Table 2-1. Summary of Early Skills for Informal Screening Evaluation

Areas of functioning	By age level: 1 year	2 years	3 years	4 years	5 years
Articulation	Babbling	Vowels; 50% intelligible	Labial consonants (b/p/m/w); 75% intelligible	Stop consonants (b/d/g/k); 95% intelligible	Fricatives (f/v/sh/ch/th); 100% intelligible
Comprehension	At least three words	At least 25 words; simple commands	Complex commands; semantic groups; many words	Large vocabulary; causal relations; simple stories	Abstractions; relationships between words; left–right
Expression	Says first word	Two-word utterances; variety of meanings; approximately 100 words	Telegraphic sentences; some morphemes	Grammatical sentences; most morphemes; approximately five-word sentences	Complex sentences; few grammar errors; can define words
Use of language	Indicates desires	Egocentric and communicative; likes stories	Announces intentions; talks a lot; takes turns talking	Describes past; egocentric language rare; likes rhyming	Learning to manipulate people with language
Play and nonverbal behavior	Plays pat-a-cake; gestures some	Uses some objects and toys correctly; scribbles	Has imaginative play	Draws objects	

sound very garbled. Mothers report that at 2 years of age, only 50% of their children's speech is intelligible whereas by 4 years of age nearly 100% is intelligible.

During the stage of systematic acquisition of speech sounds, speech dysfluency or "stuttering" may appear. This is very common in young children and seems to appear at the point in time of rapid growth in speech and language acquisition, giving rise to the popular claim that the child stutters "because his brain is working faster than his tongue." Research has shown that approximately 85% of young children who stutter during this period of time recover spontaneously in a few months' time without intervention (Homzie & Lindsay, 1984). Hence, speech pathologists generally agree that speech therapy is not indicated for young children who begin stuttering unless there is evidence of general tension, fear of talking, or avoidance of speech.

Stabilizing of Articulation Skills (50–80 Months of Age)

By the time the child is 5 years of age, approximately 90% of his utterances will be intelligible to unfamiliar adults. At 55 months of age, speech articulation is accurate for most speech sounds, with the only speech articulation errors that can be found in normal children being "lisping" (articulation errors involving the sounds /s/, /sh/, /z/, /ch/, or /dg/) or "lalling" (distortions of the sounds /l/ or /r/).

Development of Language Skills

We have seen that, prior to the time the child utters his first word, he goes through several stages of speech development; and that once the first word is uttered, the child's speech acquisition continues in an organized pattern that is grossly similar across children. The same is true of the child's language development. The basic stages of language development are discussed below.

The Prelinguistic Stage (up to 1 Year of Age)

The processes involved in language development in the young infant are extremely complex. There is increasing evidence that the young infant is aware of the sounds in his environment and is able to discriminate among them at an early age. In the first few weeks of life, the infant shows a startle response to loud or sudden sounds, and an arousal response to loud sounds during sleep. Studies have shown that an infant of 6 weeks of age can discriminate among different speech sounds.

It is generally agreed that infants communicate before they talk (Sugarman, 1983). As early as 1 month of age, the baby establishes eye contact with the parents, and by 3 months of age, the baby smiles back with the parents and laughs when talked to by the parents.

At 4 months of age, the baby typically turns his eyes and head in the direction of a source of sounds, and may change facial expressions or vocalize in response to sounds. As the baby gets older and develops better motor coordination, he begins interacting with his parents in the form of language games, such as pat-a-cake or peek-a-boo.

At approximately 6 months of age, the infant shows evidence of "selective listening," choosing to respond to some sounds and to ignore others. Between 6 and 10 months of age, the baby produces differential responses to different sounds; for example, certain sounds may cause him to vocalize, while other sounds may cause him to be quiet. Later, the baby demonstrates recognition of simple words by some action (such as pointing). Commonly first-recognized words include the baby's name, "no," and "hot." At this stage of development, the baby may begin looking at pictures being named by the mother, and listening to speech without being distracted by other sounds.

By 15 months of age, but before the first word is uttered, the toddler begins communicating by vocalizing and simultaneously pointing at desired objects. Other simple gestures—for example, tugging or staring at a person to indicate a desire, waving "bye-bye," shaking the head "no," or following in the direction of an adult's pointing—are also used for communication at this stage. It is not known whether these preverbal forms of communication are necessary prerequisites of formal language acquisition or merely precursors (Golinkoff, 1983).

The Single-Word Utterance Stage (12–18 Months of Age)

The average age when a child utters his first word is 11 months, although the range of 8–18 months is considered normal for the appearance of first words (Morley, 1965). First words are often accompanied by gestures—for example, waving and saying "bye" (to indicate "good-bye") or peeking and saying "boo" (to indicate "peek-a-boo"). Between 12 and 18 months of age, the child generally makes utterances consisting of single words. First words typically refer to items in the immediate environment, and are typically chosen from names of persons, animals, toys, foods, and activities. From within this universal set of vocabulary items, individual styles of word usage are found. For example, at the one-word utterance stage, a child may be identified as either an "expressive speaker" tending to use personal–social expressions ("whoops," "pat-a-cake"), or a "referential speaker" tending to use object names (Nelson, 1973).

Many authors propose that one-word utterances are not merely simple acts of labeling on the part of the child. Rather, single-word utterances (or "holophrastic" speech) may represent instances where the single words are used by the child to express more complex ideas. Thus, if the baby says "Mama," he may be trying to convey a more complex message such as "Mama, come here," rather than labeling or identifying his mother.

Research has, in fact, suggested that "first meanings" conveyed by infants are of two basic types: "positive volition" (e.g., saying "Mama" to indicate a desire of some type) and "negative volition" (e.g., saying "no" to indicate a refusal to do something) (Greenfield & Smith, 1976).

During the one-word utterance stage, when the child is in the process of building his vocabulary, phenomena called "underextension" and "overextension" have been observed (Nelson & Bonvillian, 1978). "Overextension" refers to the use of a word to refer to something more general or more extended than the word's "real" meaning (e.g., "doggie" to refer to any animal, or "Dada" to refer to any adult male). It has been pointed out that the child's use of "overextension" should not imply a misperception of the meaning of the word. Thus, the child who says "doggie" to label a cat may, in fact, recognize that the cat is not a "doggie," but uses that term because he lacks the other word. "Underextension" refers to the child's use of a word to signify only a part of the word's "real" meaning (e.g., the use of "car" to signify only moving cars, as distinct from parked cars).

Essentially, the process of word acquisition is one in which constant refinements and redefinitions are made by the child until his meanings correspond to the "real" adult meanings (Anglin, 1970; R. Brown, 1978; H. H. Clark, 1977). This process can take years for some words.

During the single-word stage, the child is often heard talking to himself or engaging in "egocentric speech" (Piaget, 1926). It has been observed that at this stage the child just seems to chatter away, apparently unconcerned as to whether or not there is any listener. "Self-imperatives," in which the child states what he is doing (e.g., he may say "go" as he walks along), are common.

The child does not only talk to himself in single words; he also may use jargon or long patterns of speech sounds that seem to have meaning to him, but that are not meaningful to adults. Jargon or unintelligible utterances that have conversational inflection and that appear to have meaning for the child seem to be produced by all normal children in the 18- to 22-month age range (Trantham & Pedersen, 1976).

At this time, the child's nonverbal play also shows understanding of common household objects and their functions. The child is beginning to use objects such as combs, keys, and cups appropriately.

Although the relationship between comprehension and production of words is unclear, it is generally believed that the young child is able to understand a great many more words than he is able to use in speech. By the time the child is 18 months of age, he may only be saying one or two words, but he commonly is able to understand a number of other words. The names of several body parts, household objects, toys, and family members are normally understood by an 18-month-old. At this stage, the child's attention to sounds extends to a much larger range, and the child will respond to sounds from other rooms for which there are no visual cues (for example, the sound of a refrigerator opening in another room).

The Two-Word Utterance Stage (18–24 Months of Age)

After the child begins using single words to communicate, there is a period of time in which the child builds his vocabulary of single words. Words for people, animals, toys, foods, body parts, clothing, furniture, household objects, and vehicles are acquired. When the child has acquired an expressive vocabulary of approximately 50 single words, he begins combining words into two-word messages. In some children, a transition stage has been reported between the one-word stage and the two-word stage, during which single words are produced with pauses between them in a chain-like effect (e.g., "Mommy"—"go"). More commonly, however, two-word messages with smooth, sentence-like intonation patterns appear naturally among the single-word utterances (e.g., "Mommy go").

It has been reported that children use rules for combining words into two-word utterances (Braine, 1963). That is, they do not randomly combine words, but they only combine words in certain ways. Some words may occur in either position in a two-word utterance, whereas other words have limited occurrences.

As with the single-word utterance, it has been claimed that the two-word utterance is used by the child to express a variety of meanings (H. H. Clark, 1977). For example, during the two-word utterance stage, a child was observed using the utterance "Mommy sock" in two different situations: once when his mother was putting the child's sock on him, and once when the child found his mother's sock. These utterings of "Mommy sock" are seen as representing two different types of meanings: "agent + action" and "possessor + possession."

Studies have proposed that at the two-word utterance stage, children are capable of expressing approximately 10 different types of meanings, including "agent + action" ("baby cry"), "action + object" ("hit baby"), "agent + object" ("baby toy"), "action + location" ("fall down"), "entity + location" ("Daddy home"), and "possessor + possession" ("Mommy sock").

Just as the child's ability to express meanings during the two-word utterance stage becomes more complex, so does his ability to understand meanings. At the beginning of the two-word utterance stage, the child is able to respond to simple directions and to action commands presented without gestures or visual cues (e.g., "Give me the ball," "Come here," "Sit down"). During the two-word utterance stage, both the child's basic vocabulary and his ability to understand sentence structures increase, so that by the end of the two-word utterance stage he is beginning to be able to understand complex sentences and three- or four-part commands (e.g., "When we go home, you can have some candy," "Go to the table and get the book and the toy and bring me them"). Also, during the two-word utterance stage, the child learns to understand pronouns ("him," "her," "we," "they," "you").

Although the two-word utterance stage is a period of serious work in language acquisition, it is still a period of playfulness for the child. Along with beginning to use language to ask for his needs and to make observations about the environment, the child still uses language in an egocentric way, often talking to himself in long monologues. Also, the child shows a great deal of interest in environmental sounds, music, and television theme songs, and enjoys imitating them.

The child's expressive language at this stage of development may be very perseverative. Appropriate "conversations" are rare. It is not abnormal for the child to talk perseveratively about a single topic for a long time, or to echo his own utterances or parts of the utterances of others (Fay & Anderson, 1981). Echolalia has been documented in normal children, usually between the ages of 18 and 23 months, and ceasing around the age of 27 months. This early echoing appears to be largely unselective, in contrast to later echoing, which centers primarily on unfamiliar words (Trantham & Pedersen, 1976).

At this stage, questions begin to figure more prominently

among children's utterances, with the children frequently asking questions for which they already know the answers. It has been hypothesized that children are gathering information about language, rather than about specific events. Further evidence of the "nonconversational" nature of children's language at this stage is the finding that approximately one-third of all children's utterances are not related in topic to the preceding adult utterances (Bloom, Rocissano, & Hood, 1976).

Beyond Two Words: The Simplified-Sentences Stage (24–36 Months of Age)

Although three-word utterances do, of course, appear in a child's language, there is no "three-word utterance stage" where a predominance of such utterances is found. The stage of language development where three-word utterances occur has been called the "telegraphic speech" stage because the utterances sound like telegrams. In telegraphic speech, certain types of words not essential for meaning are omitted from the utterances (e.g., "me go store," "Daddy sit chair," and "doggie in house"). The types of words that are usually omitted in telegraphic utterances include prepositions, articles, and auxiliary verbs.

After the two-word utterance stage, the average length of the child's utterances gradually increases as the child becomes capable of expressing more subtle shades of meaning. One way in which the length of children's utterances is increased at this time is through the incorporation of "morphemes" or "inflections"—that is, small units of language (not necessarily words) that express meaning. Such morphemes include the "-s" plural marker in "cats," the "-er" comparative marker in "smaller," and the "-ing" present progressive marker in "running." Research has shown that these morphemes or small units of meaning tend to be acquired by children in a fixed sequence, regardless of environmental exposure (Bellamy & Bellamy, 1970; B. B. Brown, 1973; De Villiers & De Villiers, 1973). Among the first morphemes acquired by children (usually by the age of 3 years) are the present progressive "-ing," the locative preposition "on," the locative preposition "in," and the "-s" noun plural.

Overgeneralization or overextension is common in children's usage of morphemes. When children first acquire morphemes, they tend to apply them widely, often in inappropriate environments. In this way, forms such as "he goed," "it breaked," and "I comed" are produced.

At this stage, the child begins to understand relationships and comparisons between items. He will be able to identify "the big one" versus "the little one," and he will be able to understand functional relationships ("Why do we eat?" "Why do we sleep?"). In addition, the child is beginning to recognize semantic classes (meaning groups) and knows that "Grandma" and "baby" are both "family," and that "milk" and "juice" are both "food." The child's vocabulary is growing rapidly at this stage of language development, and his use of language becomes markedly more "adult-like." Real conversations now occur with other children as well as adults, and the frequency of egocentric speech or monologues decreases. Both echoing of speech and use of nonsense jargon gradually disappear, and the child shows more communicative intent. Parents may complain that children at this stage "talk too much" and "can't be shut up." As well as talking a lot, the child at this stage wants to be heard and expects to be understood. Intentions are announced before taking action, and frustration or even tantrums occur if statements are not understood.

Grammar Development Stage (36–55 Months of Age)

The period of the most rapid development of language occurs in the child's third year of life. At this time, all aspects of language advance rapidly, with significant increases occurring in vocabulary, receptive abilities, and expressive range. The interrelationships among the ways in which the various components of language grow are not understood. It appears, however, that there is considerable variation among linguistic components and among normal children in terms of developmental changes.

Once a child's utterances become longer by virtue of more than two morphemes or words occurring in an utterance, they also become more grammatically complex. The manner in which grammar becomes more complex, while varying somewhat from child to child, does tend to follow a general pattern of development in which certain forms are always acquired before certain other forms.

The first step in grammar development includes the addition of morphemes to the two-word utterances, and expansions of single nouns and verbs into nouns and verb phrases. For example, instead of using simple one-word noun phrases (e.g., "kitty," "baby," or "doggie"), the child begins to use more complex noun phrases consisting of determiners and/or adjectives plus nouns (e.g., "that soft kitty," "my nice baby," or "his nice doggie"). Also, instead of using simple one-word verb phrases, the child uses more complex verb phrases including auxiliaries (e.g., "will" or "can"), complex verbs (e.g., "wanna go," "hafta eat," or "gonna play"), and later negatives (e.g., "don't" or "can't").

The next step in grammar development after the expansion of noun and verb phrases is the child's learning to move around the elements in a sentence in order to express new meanings. For example, the child learns to ask questions by moving the subject and object positions in a sentence ("Can we go?" instead of "We can go?") and by placing "wh-" words at the beginning of sentences ("Where is the dog?"). At this stage of development, the child masters the switching of pronouns "I" and "you" to answer questions correctly ("Are you hungry?" "Yes, I am.").

The next step in the grammar development stage involves the child's learning to combine different sentences into a single sentence by means of a process that linguists call "embedding" or "coordination." Examples of embedding include relative clauses (e.g., "The boy who is my friend is going," "I saw the car that belongs to Susie") and complement structures (e.g., "I want to go outside," "I think that I can."). Examples of coordination include sentences in which subjects are conjoined (e.g., "Mommy and Daddy eat," formed linguistically from the two sentences "Mommy eats" and "Daddy eats"), and sentences in which predicates are conjoined (e.g., "Mommy eats and drinks," "Mommy is big but weak").

During this rapid development of expressive grammatical skills, rapid development of receptive skills also occurs. Vocabulary shows its most rapid increases; studies have estimated that between the age of 3 and 4 years, the child acquires 1000 words or more. It is at this stage of development that the child masters spatial and temporal words ("under," "above," "in front of," "in back of," "behind," "between," "first," "before"), as well as concepts of cause or effect ("What do you do when you are hungry?" "Why did Mommy put on the sweater?"). Also, at this stage of development, the child is able to complete simple analogies ("Food is to eat as milk is to ______.").

The child's use of language grows more and more sophisticated at this stage of development. Egocentric use of language is extremely rare, and echolalia disappears entirely from the child's speech. While language is used to announce intentions and to describe ongoing events, there is increasing use of language to describe events and incidents from the past and to relate incidents from the past to present events. The child still enjoys "playing with language," but his forms of play become more sophisticated, and include use of rhymes, jokes, and exaggerations. The child becomes interested in being told meanings of words, is able to give reasonable definitions of words, and may enjoy hearing or even producing puns. There is a growing awareness of the "conversational" function of language, with the child being more likely to await responses and less likely to ignore interruptions than when he was younger (C. Garvey & Berninger, 1981).

Subtle Refinement of Language Abilities (55 Months of Age Onward)

By the time the child has passed his fourth birthday, his basic knowledge of his language is complete. From this time on, the rapid development of many areas of language skills is no longer seen. Language development slows down, and additions to the linguistic system take the form of subtle refinements. At times, it may appear that more complex sentence structures are lost and then regained (Wallach, 1984).

At the 5-year level, grammatical errors are less noticeable in the child's speech, and most grammatical errors are self-corrected. However, some grammatical constructions are still not fully mastered, and errors occur when the child uses these constructions. Such constructions include agreement of nouns and verbs for singular versus plural (e.g., "He haves the toy"), distinctions of mass versus count nouns (e.g., "Give me some moneys," "I want more macaronis"), pronoun case forms (e.g., "Him and her went"), past-tense irregular verb formations ("The candy had been aten," "Yesterday she drawed the picture"), pronoun deletions in sentences (e.g., "My sister, she went to school"), and prepositions of time and place ("She takes at the school").

By the age of 6 years, grammatical differences between the child's language and adult language are not apparent without more extensive probing. Syntactic formations that have not been mastered at age 6 are more complex (Barrie-Blackley, 1973; Chomsky, 1969; Palermo & Molfese, 1972). These include structures such as "The doll is easy to see" (where the child may assign "the doll" as subject of the utterance, interpreting the utterance as meaning "The doll can easily see"), "John asked Mary where to go" (where the child may not be able to determine whether it is John or Mary who is confused about where to go), and "John promised Bill to leave" (where the child may assign "Bill" as subject of the utterance, interpreting the utterance as meaning that "John promised that Bill would leave").

By the time the child reaches 8 years of age, his adult grammar should be fully formed. Additions to the linguistic system after the age of 8 years are limited to semantic items and refinements in the way in which language is used. Among the vocabulary refinements that occur are a wider understanding of concepts of number, speed, time, and spatial relationships, and a wider understanding of emotional, abstract, and figurative terms (e.g., "misery," "democracy," or "justice"). Between 8 and 12 years of age, when the child's awareness of language reaches a higher level that allows him to recognize different levels of meaning (Van Kleeck, 1984), interest in puns, jokes, and riddles becomes intense (Lodge & Leach, 1975). In addition, the child learns to categorize items into semantic classes, and to identify synonyms, antonyms, and multiple meanings of a word.

The 6-year-old child uses language to tell stories, share ideas, and discuss alternatives. The child begins to tell detailed stories linking events in an organized manner to preceding and following events. Between the ages of 6 and 12 years, the child becomes increasingly skilled at adapting the type of language he uses to the environment in which he finds himself. Polite forms, for example, increase in frequency of occurrence as the child develops a sense of their usefulness (Leonard, Schwartz, Folger, & Wilcox, 1978). While the 5-year-old child might say, "Don't play with my toys," the 7-year-old child might say, "I'd rather you didn't play with my toys." The child at this stage also develops a sense of when bartering or offering alternatives is necessary: "You can play with my toys if I can have your candy."

The ability to understand discrepancies between meaning and form in utterances increases after 5 years of age (H. Gardner, Kircher, Winner, & Parkins, 1975; Ortony, Reynolds, & Arter, 1978). For example, a 5-year-old child may think that "to pull the wool over one's eyes" means to cover someone's face, whereas the older child will recognize that the expression means "to deceive." As the child learns to move away from literal interpretations, he becomes more adept at abstract interpretations of language, such as "reading between the lines," making inferences, and interpreting unusual word orders. It is not until the teen years when discrepancies between voice and message (e.g., the sarcastic tone of voice) are appreciated.

CHAPTER 3

Assessment of Speech and Language Development

Introduction

The assessment and diagnosis of childhood speech or language deficits are often complex matters. This is partially due to the variety of manifestations of speech and language disorders that may occur.

In this volume, a distinction is made between "assessment" (the determination of functional levels in different areas) and "differential diagnosis" (the determination of a particular diagnosis); these issues are discussed throughout several chapters. The present chapter contains a general discussion of principles and techniques for assessment. A discussion of differential diagnosis of various syndromes involving speech and language is given in Chapter 4, and in Chapter 5 case illustrations are presented.

The discussion of assessment procedures that follows in the present chapter is organized into a series of decision-making steps for clinicians to use in assessing various areas of speech or language development. The discussion includes some general remarks about informal assessment, and more specific descriptions of methods for screening of deficits in different areas of speech or language development. For each of the areas covered, mention is made of those formal tests that are most appropriate for providing additional specific information. This chapter is intended primarily as a guide for clinicians who are not trained in speech or language pathology, and aims to provide an overview of the types of procedures that are used to assess various aspects of language. We hope that the chapter, by dealing with questions such as "What does it mean if a child scores poorly on a particular test?" "What do particular tests measure?" and "How do particular tests relate to particular clinical observations?", will prove helpful in the interpretation of reports from speech or language pathologists.

The assessment of speech and language development may involve either informal screening procedures or formal testing procedures. Informal procedures have the advantages of being more rapid to administer and interpret; of being more likely to elicit cooperation from very young, very shy, or very oppositional children; and of providing examples of language behaviors in relatively naturalistic settings.

In general, informal procedures are sufficient to determine the presence of any problems in speech or language development, whereas formal tests are required to provide a more specific delineation of the scope of such problems. Formal tests are also useful in providing a "map" of a child's overall strengths and weaknesses, and as an aid in formulating a treatment program or educational plan.

The informal screening procedures discussed below fall into three general types: a medical, family, and developmental history obtained from the parents; observation of the child; and semistructured interactions with the child. The history is particularly important when dealing with very young children, who may be unable or unwilling to respond to informal or formal tests, and whose behaviors during observations in the office may not be representative of their overall abilities. We have found that parents are able to provide the most reliable histories if they are probed for specific examples of behaviors, rather than if they are simply asked for yes–no or age-level responses. The use of a specific background history form (such as the one included as Appendix A to this chapter) can prove useful in enumerating points to be covered. A joint review of baby books, photo albums, or home movies can also be helpful in establishing a clear and reliable history of the child's development.

The observations of the child should ideally occur in several settings, such as in the home, at school, or at play with other children. In a clinical setting, covert observations of the child interacting with his mother or with another child are initially valuable, since they free the observer from the need for simultaneously conversing with the child. During observations, it is helpful to have at hand a chart of developmental norms (such as the one provided in Table 2-1 in the preceding chapter) and a list of symptoms (such as the one provided later in this chapter in Appendix B).

A "play" situation is best for obtaining semistructured responses from young children. The examiner should preferably seat himself on the child's level (i.e., at a low table or on the floor) surrounded by an assortment of toys, books, and common objects (e.g., keys, forks and spoons, crayons or pencils, and cups). The child can at first be left to his own devices with the toys and objects. We have found that it is most successful to begin semistructured assessments with nonverbal tasks (e.g., drawing, building with blocks, or pointing out objects in books). Then, as the child warms up, the examiner can take a more active part by encouraging the child to verbalize. More detailed information on methods of informal screening can be found in the following references: Bax, Hart, and Jenkins (1980), Capute and Accardo (1978), Carrow (1972), Fay (1980), Hixson (1979), Lynch (1979), A. H. Schwartz and Murphy (1975), and Wiig and Semel (1980).

Systematic Assessment of Specific Areas

Assessment of Responses to Sounds (Hearing Impairment, Auditory Processing)

Abnormal responses to sounds are suggestive of impairments either in hearing or in auditory processing abilities. (As we discuss in the following chapter, hearing impairments and auditory processing deficits are clinical features of a number of syndromes involving language development.)

Assessment of responses to sounds can often be done without involving the child in linguistic interactions. Thus, this type of assessment may be less threatening to the child who has had previous negative experiences associated with verbal communication. Parents may also be more comfortable when the evaluation begins with questions that appear to be directed toward hearing deficits rather than mental retardation or brain malfunction.

Assessment of responses to sounds should begin with a thorough medical and developmental history. Risk factors for hearing impairments include pregnancy, birth, and neonatal problems (e.g., high bilirubin levels, high fevers, convulsions, anoxia, Rh incompatibility, apnea, jaundice, or congenital anomalies); recurrent diseases (in particular, ear infections); serious infectious diseases (e.g., mumps, meningitis, or encephalitis); familiar disorders (family history of hearing impairment); and use of ototoxic medications (those in the mycin or quinine families).

In taking a developmental history, it may be possible to find evidence of abnormal responses to sounds dating from infancy. Parents should be questioned for examples of responses to different types of sounds at different age levels; examples of the length of the child's attention span; and examples of the types of things that most held the child's attention at different age levels. Children who have a history of no startle response to loud sounds, or no responses to household sounds (e.g., cars, vacuum cleaners, or television sets) or to human voices by the age of 1 year, are especially suspect for hearing impairment. In cases where there is any history at all suggestive of abnormal responses to sounds, the clinician should try to determine from the parents exactly what types of sounds can and cannot elicit a response from the child. It can be important if a child shows a differential response between loud versus soft sounds, between high- versus low-pitched sounds, between speech when facing versus not facing the speaker, or between voices versus environmental sounds.

In making observations of the child's responses to sounds, the clinician should think in terms of three questions: (1) "Is the child listening normally?" (2) "Is the child attending normally?" and (3) "Is the child hearing normally?" In particular, the clinician should observe the child for localizing of sounds (whether the child turns his head or gazes in the direction of sounds of different types, such as a bell ringing, a person speaking, or a knock at the door); the use of excessively loud speech; and the frequent asking of "Huh?" or "What?" Children whose medical history reveals risk factors for hearing impairment, and who by either history or observation have inconsistent or unusual responses to sounds, should be referred for audiological evaluation.

It is important to remember that abnormal responses to sounds are not always indicative of hearing impairment. One example is the child who is constantly asking "What?" or "Huh?" and who seems to suffer hearing loss. It has been our experience that such a child often has normal hearing, but a deficit in either listening or perceiving. (The assessment of such deficits is discussed below in "Assessment of Auditory Processing.")

Assessment of Receptive Language (Grammar and Vocabulary)

Another area of assessment requiring nonverbal responses from the child is the child's comprehension of language.

Although parental reports of language development are usually reliable, we have found that the area of language comprehension is one of the least reliable aspects of the speech and language history. There may be gross overestimates of a child's abilities, due to the fact that the child may respond appropriately to instructions because of situational cues, nonverbal cues, or chance, rather than because of true linguistic comprehension of a command. The language scales or language screening tests (tests 48 and 66 in Appendix C) that use information from parental interviews may be similarly unreliable. However, for very young or uncooperative children, these scales may be the only way of collecting any information.

For older children, there are three general methods of informally assessing language comprehension: (1) asking a child to identify objects or pictures, (2) asking the child to follow commands, (3) and asking the child to act out utterances using dolls or toys. All of these methods separate language comprehension and expression skills by requiring a nonverbal response from the child.

In creating an informal test for language comprehension, tasks involving increasing levels of complexity should be given. For example, the child can first be asked to point out objects or body parts as they are named (e.g., "Where's the doggie?"); then to show activities (e.g., "Show me 'running'"); then to respond to one-part, two-part, and three-part commands (e.g., "Give me the book," "Sit down and close the book," "Stand up, clap your hands, and then turn around"); and finally to carry out actions with dolls or toys (e.g., "Make the girl hit the boy").

In order to judge accurately whether a child has comprehended a command, the clinician must be very careful to avoid giving nonverbal cues to the child. The command "Give me the toy car" when accompanied by an open palm or a gaze toward the toy can be rapidly carried out by a child who has no idea what any of the words may mean. Research has shown that informal assessment procedures are less reliable in determining language comprehension levels than in determining other levels of language functioning, because of the variety of nonlinguistic strategies that children can use to decode commands (R. Chapman, 1978; Oviatt, 1980). Therefore, tasks for comprehension assessment should involve unusual rather than usual instructions (e.g., "Kiss the book" rather than "Open the book").

There are a number of good tests of language comprehension available, some testing the comprehension of vocabulary items, and some testing the comprehension of grammatical items. Both types of tests are necessary since, particularly in the case of older children, there may be a discrepancy between vocabulary comprehension and grammatical or "linguistic" comprehension.

Tests 27, 42, and 64 in Appendix C measure the comprehension of vocabulary items. Of these, test 42 (the Peabody Picture Vocabulary Test) is the most reliable and comprehensive, having been recently revised and normed for all age groups from 2 years through adult.

Tests of grammatical comprehension require either that the child select a picture representing a particular grammatical structure, or that the child perform actions to indicate knowledge of the structures. The structures examined vary according to the age of the child being tested, but typically include items such as different verb tenses, temporal and spatial concepts ("before," "after," "under," "over"), and linguistic delimiters ("all . . . except," "if . . . then").

Tests 12 and 13 in Appendix C (the "processing" subtests) are generally recommended for all school-aged children. For younger children (below 7 years), additional recommended tests are: those in Appendix C numbered 2, 40 (the "receptive" portion), 58, and 62 (the "grammatic understanding" subtest). For intermediate-age-level children (7–12 years), tests 62 (the "grammatic understanding" subtest) and 63 are recommended. And for children above the age of 12 years, test 17 (the "oral directions" and "oral commissions" subtests) is recommended.

Children coming from bilingual language backgrounds should additionally be tested in the other language. Recommended tests that cover corresponding receptive language skills in both English and Spanish are those numbered 15 and 58.

Assessment of Speech Production (Articulation, Fluency, Intonation, and Voice)

As will be seen later, abnormalities in speech development are features of a variety of syndromes, including developmental language disorder, developmental articulation disorder, hearing impairment, and pervasive developmental disorders.

The assessment of speech development begins with a developmental history covering the child's vocalizations and oral behaviors, and a social history covering psychosocial factors associated with delayed speech development. The psychosocial risk factors include low socioeconomic status (as determined by parental education and occupation), large family size, late birth order, twinship, and bilingual background.

Early vocalizations that are described as being uneven in pitch, or of extremely shrill pitch, are suggestive of abnormality. The absence of any vocalizations or imitations of sounds by the age of 6 months, the absence of any babbling involving consonant sounds by the age of 1 year, or a history of speech that is less than 50% intelligible by 3 years of age are clearly abnormal. A history of no noticeable increase in speech clarity over a 6-month period for children between the ages of 1 and 4 years is also abnormal. Speech that is reported to be usually or always hoarse, congested, nasal, or whiny is abnormal and suggestive of organic involvement, as is a history of problems in chewing, sucking, or swallowing.

In order to obtain the most objective history possible, it is useful to ask whether, at a particular age, other adults who were not family members could understand the child; whether the child was ever teased about his speech by other children; and whether the child's nursery teachers ever commented that the child seemed behind other children his age in speech development.

Speech assessment should include observation of the child's speech and articulation skills, examination of the oral speech mechanism for deformities, and informal testing of oral motor skills by asking the child to imitate various oral motor activities (e.g., sticking out the tongue, "chattering" with the teeth, blowing, or producing certain syllables).

In observing the child's speech and articulation skills, the following should be noted: apparent embarrassment or avoidance of speech; apparent struggle to speak (e.g., grimaces, blinks, or frowns); drooling; misordering of speech sounds; repetitions of words or speech sounds; and speech that is abnormally fast or slow. In addition, an estimate of the overall intelligibility of the child's speech is useful. Formal articulation assessment consists of observing the inventory of speech sounds that the child can correctly produce, and comparing this inventory to the "norms" for the child's age.

The tests available to assess articulation skills consist of naming or imitation procedures, and are a useful way of rapidly eliciting an inventory of speech sounds in a variety of positions in words. Recommended articulation tests include those in Appendix C numbered 1, 6, 16, and 29. Unfortunately, no formal tests are available for assessing voice, fluency, or intonation skills, and the development of these skills must be assessed largely by impression.

Assessment of Expressive Language (Grammar and Vocabulary)

Although the assessment of expressive language consists primarily of getting the child to talk, there are certain family and developmental factors that should be covered in the history with the parents. These are the presence of a family history of speech, language, or learning disorders; the number and ages of family members and how much time they spend talking with the child; the languages that the child has been exposed to; the amount of time the child is away from the home; the nature and quality of alternative care arrangements; and the ages and language backgrounds of any playmates the child may have.

A basic history of expressive language development includes milestones (such as first word and first sentence) and a general description of how the child communicated at various age levels, including the manner of communication (e.g., vocalizations, gestures, or combinations of vocalizations and gestures) and the "triggers" for communication (e.g., whether the child communicated only with certain people, only at certain times of the day, or only in order to achieve certain goals). In addition, a description of any observed expressive language problems (e.g., difficulty learning new words, remembering words, or putting words together into sentences) should be obtained.

Observations of the child in a naturalistic conversational setting should be made, with particular attention to errors in vocabulary or word usage, the typical length of the child's utterances, and the variety of grammatical forms used. Other aspects of expressive language to observe include pauses of inordinate length before responses, numerous revisions or self-interruptions, difficulty with word finding, and excessive use of overgeneralized words (e.g., "this," "that," "it," "thing," "stuff," or "these").

In instances where it is not possible to elicit a naturalistic speech sample, it may be necessary to manipulate the environment in order to obtain a sample of the child's language. One such method of manipulating the environment in order to produce a language sample is by having the child play with toys, books, or other children, and by simultaneously asking the child general questions such as "Tell me what you are doing." Following the more general questions, the child can be probed for specific linguistic items (e.g., names of objects, functions of objects, locatives, or possessives). In cases of children with moderate or severe expressive deficits, comparing the output to a table of general language norms (such as Table 2-1) will immediately reveal deficits. However, systematic linguistic analysis may be necessary to reveal more subtle deficits. One such method is Developmental Sentence Analysis (DSA; Lee, 1974), which provides a technique for analyzing a sample of utterances for grammatical complexity.

Sentence imitation is a technique that is particularly useful for eliciting a sample of expressive output from children who are very shy or quiet. This approach is based upon the experimental evidence that children are not able to repeat grammatical structures that they cannot themselves spontaneously produce (Wiig & Semel, 1980). In this approach, the clinician (or the child's mother, if necessary) produces a series of increasingly longer and more complex utterances, asking the child to repeat each one. The types of sentences and words that the child accurately imitates are noted. Children under the age of 8 years with developmental language disorder are generally unable to imitate sentences longer than three or four words.

There are a number of normed tests of sentence imitation that are useful. These include tests 11, 12 (the "model sentences" subtest), 15, 17 (the "auditory attention span for related syllables"), 40 (the "expressive" portion), 59 (the "sentence repetition" subtest), and 62 (the "sentence imitation" subtest) in Appendix C.

For older children who have more language and who are more cooperative, expressive language can be informally tested by having the child describe a television show plot, paraphrase a story, define words, or fill in the blanks in a mutual story-telling situation. Specific grammatical structures can be elicited by the use of carrier phrases (e.g., "This one is big, but that one is . . . ") and nonsense items (e.g., "This is a wug, and these are two . . . "). Recommended formal tests for children in the 3- to 12-year age group include those numbered 12 and 13 (the various "production" subtests), 23, 35 (the "grammatic closure" and "verbal expression" subtests), 45 (the "verbal" subtests), and 62 (the "oral vocabulary" and "grammatic closure" subtests) in Appendix C.

More advanced children might be asked to identify similarities and differences, explain the functions of items, or complete analogies. Recommended tests of expressive language for children above the age of 11 years include numbers 12 and 13 (the "production" subtests), 28, and 52 (the "vocabulary" and "proverb explanation" subtests).

Assessment of Auditory Processing

ASSESSMENT OF SKILLS IN AUDITORY ATTENTION

Auditory processing can only be reliably assessed in older verbal children. Attempts to assess auditory processing using observations or informal testing methods are often inadequate, since dysfunctions in processing may be rather subtle.

Nonetheless, there are several techniques that can be used informally to attempt to isolate areas of auditory processing dysfunctions. We have found the game "Simon Says" to be useful in indicating auditory attention or concentration problems, as well as problems in auditory discrimination or memory. Children with attention deficit disorder typically fail to produce the differential responses between the "Simon Says" and distractor instructions. A good screening test for younger children that uses the "Simon Says" format is test 13 in Appendix C. Two other tests of auditory attention aimed at somewhat older children are tests 25 and 30.

ASSESSMENT OF SKILLS IN AUDITORY DISCRIMINATION

A simple screening for auditory discrimination deficits involves saying minimal pairs of words (different in only one sound, such as "bat, pat"; "tan, tam") and asking the child if the words are the same or different. Such an approach requires that the child understand the meanings not only of the words presented, but also of the concepts "same" and "different." Furthermore, caution must be used when presenting the stimulus words not to give away any difference between the words by using a pattern of contrastive stress when saying the word pairs.

There are several formal screening tests for auditory discrimination available. Among those recommended are tests 3, 10, 13, 32, and 62 in Appendix C. There are several other tests for auditory discrimination that are more complex in format and have limited clinical usefulness, including tests 21, 51, 53, and 54.

ASSESSMENT OF SKILLS IN AUDITORY MEMORY

Tasks such as repeating strings of digits, words, or sentences can reveal deficits in auditory memory. On such tasks, a differential performance in repeating nonsense versus real words, or strings of unrelated words versus sentences, can be indicative of specific language dysfunction. Differential performance in repetition between auditorily presented stimuli and visually presented stimuli is also significant.

A number of tests of sentence repetition are mentioned in "Assessment of Expressive Language," above. Tests 5, 35 (the "auditory sequential memory" subtest), and 67 in Appendix C assess auditory memory for digits ("digit span"). Tests 4 and 7 (the "auditory attention span for unrelated words" subtest) assess auditory memory for unrelated words.

A number of the formal tests designed to assess language comprehension also assess auditory memory to a certain extent, since their structure requires that the child "hold in mind" an auditory presentation and then act on it. Those tests of comprehension that are structured with a series of commands of controlled lengths provide the best clues to auditory memory as separated from language comprehension. Recommended tests of this type include tests 2 and 63.

ASSESSMENT OF SKILLS IN OTHER AREAS OF AUDITORY PROCESSING: "SOUND BLENDING," AUDITORY CLOSURE, AND AUDITORY ASSOCIATION

"Sound blending" refers to the ability of the child to put together strings of sounds into words. This is usually tested by presenting "broken-up" words (such as "u-p," "c-a-t," or "m-ilk") and asking the child to say the words at a normal rate. Among the formal tests that assess sound blending are tests 8, 31, 35 (the "sound blending" subtest), and 50 in Appendix C. "Auditory association" refers to the ability of the child to associate and remember sound-to-symbol pairing. Tests that aim to assess auditory association include 31, 35 (the "auditory association" subtest), and 38. "Auditory closure" refers to the ability to fill in the blanks in a partially heard auditory signal. Test 35 (the "auditory closure" subtest) measures this ability, as do some of the tests of auditory discrimination (discussed above) that use masking.

Assessment of "Pragmatics": Language Usage and Thought Disorder

"Pragmatics," or how the child uses language to communicate, can provide information needed in making diagnoses of thought disorder, as well as of various types of language disorder. The assessment of pragmatics must involve observations, since there are no standardized tests available to assess this feature of language development.

In observing a child for features of language use, it is necessary to be aware of the purposes for which the child uses language (e.g., to ask questions, to make spontaneous remarks, or to issue commands). Both nonverbal and verbal features of language and communication are involved. Although the speech sample should ideally be obtained in a naturalistic conversational setting, we have found that deficits in pragmatic functioning can usually be discovered in the clinical setting. Table 3-1 lists the verbal and nonverbal features that are suggestive of pragmatic deficits in children. The presence of any of these features in the child's interactions should be noted. The Scale for the Assessment of Thought, Language, and Communication by Andreasen (1979) provides a list of features that have been found to be associated with pragmatic and thought disorders in adults, but this scale is less readily applicable for use with the children. A more detailed discussion of this scale may be found in Chapter 4.

Table 3-1. Features of Pragmatic Deficits

Verbal Features
1. Poor topic maintenance—rapid and inappropriate changes of topic with no transitional cues for the listener; no "turn taking."
2. Limited verbal output—few spontaneous utterances; very rapid speech; prods and encouragement to speak.
3. Excessive verbal output—many spontaneous utterances; very rapid speech; hard to "get a word in edgewise."
4. Inappropriate use of language—utterances that are grammatically correct, but that convey semantically bizarre or inappropriate information.
5. Undergeneralization—use of very narrow word meanings; personalized or concrete examples; specific rather than general statements.
6. Echolalia—immediate repetitions of own or other person's utterances with no communicative function.
7. Delayed echolalia—use of utterances that were apparently heard previously and are repeated verbatim.
8. Egocentric speech—utterances in which the child is apparently "talking to himself."
9. Perseveration—continuing references to earlier topics or responses.
10. Jargon—use of "nonwords" (nonmeaningful phonetic strings) that have apparent personal meaning for the child.
11. Neologisms—use of utterances or words whose meaning is idiosyncratic to the child.
12. Pronoun reversals—confusions of the pronouns "I" or "me" with "you."
Nonverbal features
1. Facial expressiveness—affect and facial expressions inappropriate to the semantic content of the child's speech.
2. Gaze avoidance—consistent lack of eye contact during communication.
3. Laughter—inappropriate laughter; excessive "nervous" laughter.
4. Uncooperativeness—refusal to cooperate in play or testing; crying; showing overt lack of interest or hostile behaviors, such as hitting, spitting, etc.

Assessment of Nonlanguage Developmental Levels (Motor Skills, Performance Intelligence, "Inner Language," and Visual Processing)

In order to establish the presence of a specific impairment of linguistic functions, assessment of the nonlanguage developmental skills of the child is necessary. This is of particular importance with regard to establishing a diagnosis of mental retardation.

The general developmental factors to be covered in the history include developmental milestones (e.g., ages of smiling, sitting, standing, and walking) and a general description of developmental behaviors (e.g., the presence of abnormal developmental behaviors such as rocking, twirling, or flapping; the types of play activities at different ages; and the general activity levels of the child over time). It is useful to determine when and if random play (e.g., sucking or pounding objects), explorative play (e.g., manipulating objects), functional play (e.g., using objects appropriately), creative play (e.g., using a box as a house), and imaginative play (e.g., "cops and robbers") occurred.

During observation, an estimate can be made of the child's general maturity, play, and developmental level, and the presence of a highly developed communication system of signs or gestures should be noted.

A number of tests are available for assessing nonverbal developmental skills. These include tests of visual processing (visual memory, visual discrimination, and visual closure), such as the appropriate subtests of tests 17, 35, 45, and 67 in Appendix C, and tests of nonverbal intelligence, such as the nonverbal sections of tests 69 and 70.

Appendix A. Background History Questionnaire

Pregnancy, Birth, Neonatal

Is there any history of:
____ jaundice and/or an abnormally high bilirubin level?
____ anoxia?
____ Rh incompatibility?
____ apnea?
____ congenital anomalies?

Childhood Illnesses

Has/have there ever been any:
____ high fever?

____ febrile seizures?
____ convulsions?
____ recurrent ear infections?
____ infectious diseases (mumps, scarlet fever, rubella, meningitis, or encephalitis)?
____ use of ototoxic drugs (mycins, quinine)?

Family History

Is there any family history of:
____ hearing impairment?
____ speech or language impairment?
____ learning difficulties?
____ genetic disorders?

What is/are:
____ the paternal educational and occupational levels?
____ the maternal educational and occupational levels?
____ the family size?
____ the birth order of the target child?
____ the language background of the child (whether bilingual)?
____ amount and type of interactions child typically receives?

Appendix B. Speech and Language Checklist

Hearing Checklist

____ The child shows no startle response to loud noise.
____ The child ignores environmental sounds (cars, vacuum cleaners, television, radio, noise-making toys).
____ The child responds to loud sounds, but not soft ones.
____ The child responds to high-pitched sounds, but not low-pitched ones.
____ The child responds to speech when he is facing the person speaking, but not when he is not facing the person speaking.
____ The child responds to environmental sounds, but not voices.
____ The child's voice is usually too loud.
____ The child frequently asks "Huh?" or "What?"

Speech Checklist: Articulation

____ It is difficult for the parents or family members to understand the child's speech.

____ It is difficult for nonfamily members to understand the child's speech.
____ The child omits certain sounds from his speech. (*Example*: says "ca" instead of "car.")
____ The child substitutes certain sounds for other sounds. (*Example*: says "wabbit" instead of "rabbit.")
____ The child reverses the order of sounds within words. (*Example*: says "aminal" instead of "animal.")
____ The child has trouble saying these sounds: /s/, /sh/, or /z/.
____ The child has trouble saying these sounds: /r/, /l/, or /th/.
____ The child has trouble saying other speech sounds.
____ The child often makes nonspeech vocalizations, (*Examples*: screams, hums, clicks tongue.)
____ The child has something wrong with his mouth. (*Examples*: cleft palate, weak muscles.)
____ The child has difficulty performing oral movements. (*Examples*: chewing, yawning, blowing out a match, sticking out his tongue.)
____ The child says single words correctly, but has trouble saying these same words when they occur in sentences.

Speech Checklist: Fluency and Voice

____ The child's voice is continually congested or nasal-sounding.
____ The child's voice is continually harsh-sounding.
____ The child's voice is continually breathy-sounding.
____ The child's voice is continually hoarse.
____ The child's voice is usually too soft.
____ The child speaks in a sing-song voice.
____ The child speaks in a monotone.
____ The child speaks too fast.
____ The child speaks too slowly.
____ The child's voice pitch is unusual (too high, too low).
____ The child has an unusual pattern of stressing words in sentences.
____ The child seems embarrassed about his speech.
____ The child appears to be struggling to say words. (*Examples*: makes faces, grimaces, blinks eyes, or clenches fists when talking.)

Language Checklist: Vocabulary and Concepts

____ The child misnames items, using related but incorrect words. (*Example*: "I hurt my finger" when he means "thumb.")

____ The child's vocabulary is limited, compared to other children of the same age.

____ The child overuses nonspecific vocabulary. (*Examples*: uses words like "this," "that," "thing," "stuff," "you know" instead of object names.)

____ The child uses made-up words that only he understands.

____ The child has a problem understanding concepts (particularly spatial concepts, temporal concepts, comparisons, or relationships).

____ The child can know a word one day and the next day it will be forgotten.

____ The child doesn't talk much—one has to "drag information out of him."

____ The child is unable to recognize that words can have more than one meaning.

____ The child is unable to understand figurative language, puns, idioms, or proverbs.

Language Checklist: Grammatical Rules, Language Structure, and Auditory Processing

____ The child frequently begins sentences with "um" or "uh."

____ The child mixes up the order of words in sentences.

____ The child often starts over in the middle of a sentence.

____ The child leaves out words from his sentences ("telegram-like speech").

____ The child uses grammatical forms incorrectly for his age level. (*Examples*: refers to himself as "me," as in "me want a drink"; uses simple plurals incorrectly, as in "I have three toy"; uses irregular plurals incorrectly, as in "I have two foots"; uses past-tense forms incorrectly, as in "I throwed a ball.")

____ The child pauses an excessively long time before answering questions.

____ The child fails to give significant information. (*Example*: when asked a question, will say something vague about the topic, but will not provide a satisfactory answer.)

____ The child speaks in shorter sentences compared to other children of the same age.

____ The child has difficulty telling a story in a logical, meaningful manner.

____ The child has difficulty relating facts. (*Examples*: expresses ideas in an incomplete or scattered manner; confuses the order of items; does not maintain the correct verb tenses across sentences.)

____ The child usually speaks in grammatically simple sentences.
____ The child has difficulty following verbal directions.
____ The child has difficulty understanding relationships in complex sentences.
____ The child has trouble remembering and repeating information.
____ The child has a problem expressing himself.
____ The child has a learning problem.
____ The child has difficulty attending to auditory information.
____ The child has difficulty discriminating between similar words.
____ The child has difficulty remembering (and/or repeating) things he has heard.

Language Checklist: Pragmatics and Language Use

____ The child talks to himself.
____ The child talks too much.
____ The child says bizarre or inappropriate things.
____ The child speaks in long, rambling sentences.
____ The child's speech style is inappropriate for his age level. (*Example*: frequent whining or tantrums, particularly when asked for verbal responses.)
____ The child talks continually about a certain topic, and even if someone changes the topic to something different, he insists on going back to his original topic.
____ The child repeats himself ("echoes").
____ The child repeats other people's utterances.
____ The child responds with a lot of giggling or nervous laughter when asked questions.
____ The child seems unable to recognize the use for social rules (such as politeness, greetings, farewells, general poise).
____ The child does not use language for a variety of functions (such as asking for things, asking questions, telling stories).

Appendix C. List and Description of Formal Tests

1. Arizona Articulation Proficiency Scale (Fudala, 1974)
   Areas tested (speech and language): Speech articulation
   For ages: 3–11 years
   Rating: Fair to good
   Format of test: Naming

2. Assessment of Children's Language Comprehension (ACLC) (Foster, Giddan, & Stark, 1973)
   Areas tested (speech and language): Comprehension of language
   Areas tested (processing): Auditory memory (language)
   For ages: 3–7 years
   Rating: Fair to poor
   Format of test: Child must point to picture that represents the stimulus item read by the examiner. Stimuli include single words and two-, three-, or four-word utterances.
3. Auditory Discrimination Test (Wepman, 1973)
   Areas tested (processing): Auditory discrimination (speech sounds in words)
   For ages: 5–8 years
   Rating: Fair
   Format of test: Examiner reads pairs of words that are the same or which differ by only one sound, and the child must state whether the pairs are the same or different.
4. Auditory Pointing Test (Fudala, Kunze, & Ross, 1974)
   Areas tested (processing): Auditory memory for words
   For ages: 5.0–10.11 years
   Rating: Fair to poor
   Format of test: Child must point to the picture representing the stimulus word presented.
5. Auditory Sequential Memory Test (Wepman, & Morency, 1975)
   Areas tested (processing): Memory for digit sequences
   For ages: 5–8 years
   Rating: Fair
   Format of test: Child must repeat strings of digits read by the examiner.
6. Austin Spanish Articulation Test (ASAT) (Carrow, 1974a)
   Areas tested (speech and language): Speech articulation
   For ages: 4 through 7 years
   Rating: Fair to good
   Format of test: Naming of words in Spanish.
7. Bankson Language Screening Test (Bankson, 1977)
   Areas tested (speech and language): Expressive and receptive language
   Areas tested (processing): Visual discrimination and matching; auditory memory and discrimination
   For ages: 4–8 years
   Rating: Fair to good
   Format of test: Subtests in five general categories, including (1) semantics, in which the child must point to pictures and label objects, functions, colors, and opposites; (2) morphology, in which the child must complete sentences with missing words;

(3) syntax, in which the child must complete sentences with missing words and must repeat sentences; (4) visual perception, in which the child must match pictures; and (5) auditory perception, in which the child must repeat sentences and strings of words.

8. Basic Concept Inventory (Englemann, 1967)
Areas tested (speech and language): Language comprehension
Areas tested (processing): Auditory memory (sentences), sound blending
For ages: Not normed; aimed for ages preschool to 10 years
Rating: Poor
Format of test: Three subtests: (1) The child must point to the picture that best represents the stimulus item read by the examiner; (2) the child must repeat sentences and answer yes–no questions on the sentences; (3) the child must repeat digits, interpret "unblended" words (e.g., "m-ilk"), and repeat patterns of motor activities.
9. Boehm Test of Basic Concepts (Boehm, 1971)
Areas tested (speech and language): Comprehension of space, time, quantity, and other concepts
For ages: Kindergarten to second grade
Rating: Fair
Format of test: Child must mark answer sheet to show which picture best represents the stimulus sentence read by the examiner.
10. Boston University Speech Sound Discrimination Test (Pronovost, 1953)
Areas tested (processing): Discrimination of speech sounds
For ages: Kindergarten and first grade
Rating: Poor
Format of test: Pictures of three words differing by only one sound are provided, and the child must point to the picture representing the stimulus word read by the examiner.
11. Carrow Elicited Language Inventory (CELI) (Carrow, 1974)
Areas tested (speech and language): Expressive language
Areas tested (processing): Auditory memory (sentences)
For ages: 3–8 years
Rating: Good
Format of test: Child must repeat sentences of varying complexity read by the examiner.
12. Clinical Evaluation of Language Functions: Diagnostic Battery (CELF) (Semel & Wiig, 1980a)
Areas tested (speech and language): Receptive and expressive language

Areas tested (processing): Processing words and sentences
For ages: Kindergarten through 12th grade
Rating: Good
Format of test: Thirteen subtests with various tasks, including (1) pointing to pictures representing stimulus sentences ("processing word & sentence structure"); (2) selecting the word that does not belong in a group of words ("processing word classes"); (3) answering questions involving linguistic concepts; (4) answering yes/no relational questions ("processing relationships"); (5) carrying out directions ("processing linguistic concepts/oral directions"); (6) answering questions about a paragraph read aloud by the examiner ("processing spoken paragraphs"); (7) producing word lists ("producing word series"); (8) naming color/shape combinations ("producing names on confrontation"); (9) naming words in classes ("producing word associations"); (10) sentence imitation ("producing model sentences"); (11) sentence production ("producing formulated sentences"); (12) identifying same/different words ("processing speech sounds); (13) producing target words ("producing speech sounds").

13. Clinical Evaluation of Language Functions: Screening Test (CELF) (Semel & Wiig, 1980b)
Areas tested (speech and language): Receptive and expressive language
Areas tested (processing): Auditory memory (sentences and words)
For ages: Kindergarten through 12th grade
Rating: Good
Format of test: Two subtests: (1) carrying out directions; (2) answering questions, and repeating words and sentences.

14. Deep Test of Articulation (E. T. McDonald, 1964)
Areas tested (speech and language): Speech articulation
For ages: Not normed
Rating: Fair
Format of test: Spontaneous production of limited number of sounds

15. Del Rio Language Screening Test English/Spanish (Toronto, Leverman, Hanna, Rosenzweig, & Maldonado, 1975)
Areas tested (speech and language): Receptive and expressive language, English and Spanish
Areas tested (processing): Memory for sentences
For ages: 3–7 years
Rating: Good
Format of test: Five subtests, including (1) pointing to pictures that represent words; (2) repeating sentences of varying lengths; (3) repeating sentences of varying grammatical complexities;

(4) carrying out commands; and (5) answering questions about a story.

16. Denver Articulation Screening Exam (DASE) (Drumwright, 1971)
Areas tested (speech and language): Speech articulation
For ages: 2.5 through 6 years
Rating: Fair
Format of test: Imitation of words
17. Detroit Tests of Learning Aptitude (DTLA) (H. J. Baker & Leland, 1967)
Areas tested (speech and language): Expression and comprehension
Areas tested (processing): Auditory memory (for words and sentences) and visual memory (for pictures of designs and letters)
For ages: 3–19 years
Rating: Fair to good
Format of test: Various subtests, including expressing what is wrong with nonsense pictures and sentences ("pictorial/verbal absurdities"); carrying out directions with actions or writing ("oral commissions," "oral directions"); repeating sentences or strings of words ("auditory attention span for related syllables and for unrelated words"); giving opposites; answering relational questions ("orientation"); answering information questions ("social adjustment"); and explaining why pairs of words are similar and dissimilar.
18. Development and Disorders of Written Language: The Picture Story Language Test (Myklebust, 1965)
Areas tested (speech and language): Written (expressive) language
Areas tested (processing): Association and motor coordination
For ages: School age
Rating: Fair
Format of test: The child is presented with a picture and asked to write a story about it.
19. Developmental Articulation Test (Hejna, 1968)
Areas tested (speech and language): Speech articulation
For ages: Not normed
Rating: Fair
Format of test: Naming
20. Developmental Sentence Analysis (DSA) (Lee, 1974)
Areas tested (speech and language): Expressive language
For ages: 2–6.11 years
Rating: Good
Format of test: A spontaneous sample of 100 utterances of the child is analyzed for grammatical complexity.

21. Differentiation of Auditory Perception Skills (DAPS) (Reagan & Cunningham, 1976)
Areas tested (processing): Auditory discrimination and memory for environmental sounds
For ages: Not normed, but geared to ages 5–8 years
Rating: Poor
Format of test: There are several subtests for screening of auditory perception, including forward and backward reproduction of patterns of rhythms; determining "same" or "different" for words varying for rhythmic patterns; decoding of sentences in which consonants have been omitted; and completing sentences containing analogies.
22. Environmental Language Inventory (J. D. McDonald, 1978)
Areas tested (speech and language): Expressive language
Areas tested (processing): Auditory memory (sentences)
For ages: Not normed
Rating: Fair
Format of test: The examiner carries out various actions with toys, then asks the child, "What happened?" The examiner then states what happened, with the child being expected to repeat the sentence.
23. Expressive One-Word Picture Vocabulary Test (M. F. Gardner, 1979)
Areas tested (speech and language): Expressive vocabulary
For ages: 3–12 years
Rating: Good
Format of test: The child must name picture stimuli.
24. Fisher–Logemann Test of Articulation Competence (Fisher & Logemann, 1971)
Areas tested (speech and language): Speech articulation
For ages: Not normed
Rating: Fair
Format of test: Naming and sentence production
25. Flowers Auditory Test of Selective Attention (Flowers, 1975)
Areas tested (processing): Auditory attention
For ages: Not normed; designed for school-age level
Rating: Fair
Format of test: The child must listen to a tape and mark an answer sheet to indicate if a particular word has occurred in the stimulus sentences.
26. Flowers–Costello Test of Central Auditory Abilities (Flowers, Costello, & Small, 1970)
Areas tested (speech and language): Comprehension

Areas tested (processing): Auditory attention (speech vs. background noise)
For ages: Kindergarten to sixth grade
Rating: Poor
Format of test: Stimulus utterances are presented on tape with competing speech. The child must point to items in a book that represent the stimulus utterances.

27. Full Range Picture Vocabulary Test (Ammons & Ammons, 1958)
Areas tested (speech and language): Receptive vocabulary
For ages: 2 years through adult
Rating: Good
Format of test: Child must point to the picture that represents the stimulus word read by the examiner.

28. Fullerton Language Test for Adolescents (Thorum, 1980)
Areas tested (speech and language): Language comprehension and expression; concepts and idioms
Areas tested (processing): Sound blending
For ages: 11–18 years
Rating: Fair to good
Format of test: Various subtests, including following commands; defining words; naming words in classes; syllabifying words; and defining idioms.

29. Goldman–Fristoe Test of Articulation (GFTA) (Goldman & Fristoe, 1972)
Areas tested (speech and language): Speech articulation
For ages: 1st through 12th grades (6 years and above)
Rating: Good
Format of test: Naming pictures presented

30. Goldman–Fristoe–Woodcock Auditory Selective Attention Test (Goldman, Fristoe, & Woodcock, 1976)
Areas tested (processing): Auditory memory
For ages: 3–12 years
Rating: Good
Format of test: The child must point to the picture of the stimulus word presented. Stimuli are "masked" with various types of noise (voice, fan-like noise, cafeteria noise).

31. Goldman–Fristoe–Woodcock Sound Symbol Test (Goldman, Fristoe, & Woodcock, 1974)
Areas tested (processing): Auditory recall, blending, and association
For ages: 3–12 years
Rating: Fair
Format of test: There are a variety of subtests, with tasks including the imitation of nonsense syllables; recognition of sounds in a

word; synthesizing of sounds into words; recalling associations between nonsense words and symbols; reading; and spelling.

32. Goldman–Fristoe–Woodcock Test of Auditory Discrimination (Goldman, Fristoe, & Woodcock, 1970)
    Areas tested (processing): Auditory discrimination
    For ages: 3 years to adult
    Rating: Fair to good
    Format of test: The child is trained on certain vocabulary items and then is presented with four pictures representing words that differ by a single sound. The task is to point to the picture that represents the stimulus word presented.
33. Hiskey–Nebraska Test of Learning Aptitude (H-NTLA) (Hiskey, 1966)
    Areas tested (processing): Nonverbal intelligence
    For ages: 3–16 years (for deaf or hearing-impaired children)
    Rating: Fair
    Format of test: Subtests include bead patterns; memory for color; picture identification; pictorial associations; paper folding; visual attention span; block patterns; drawing completion; memory for digits; puzzle blocks; picture analogies; and spatial reasoning. All instructions are given in pantomime.
34. Houston Test for Language Development (Crabtree, 1963)
    Areas tested (speech and language): General measure
    For ages: 6 months to 6 years
    Rating: Poor
    Format of test: Consists of two parts: (1) observation scales (for children up to 3 years of age) and (2) various tasks, including naming, drawing, counting, and answering questions.
35. Illinois Test of Psycholinguistic Abilities (ITPA) (Kirk, McCarthy, & Kirk, 1968)
    Areas tested (speech and language): Reception and expression
    Areas tested (processing): Auditory and visual memory, closure, reception, association, and sound blending
    For ages: 2–10 years
    Rating: Fair to good
    Format of test: Twelve subtests with various tasks: (1) child must answer simple yes/no questions ("auditory reception"); (2) child must identify similar pictures ("visual reception"); (3) child must supply missing word in analogies ("auditory association"); (4) child must select pictures of associated items ("visual association"); (5) child must define items ("verbal expression"); (6) child must use gestures to show the use of objects ("manual expression"); (7) child must supply missing word in sentences ("gram-

matic closure"); (8) child must find hidden objects in pictures ("visual closure"); (9) child must deduce incomplete words ("auditory closure"); (10) child must repeat strings of digits ("auditory sequential memory"); (11) child must reproduce strings of symbols ("visual sequential memory"); and (12) child must deduce words formed from strings of sounds ("sound blending").

36. Language Facility Test (Dailey, 1977)
Areas tested (speech and language): Expressive language, general measure
For ages: 2–15 years
Rating: Poor
Format of test: The child is shown sets of pictures, and is asked to tell a story about the pictures. Scoring criteria are very vague.

37. Language Proficiency Test (LPT) (Gerard & Weinstock, 1981)
Areas tested (speech and language): Receptive and expressive language
Areas tested (processing): Reading and writing
For ages: Ninth grade to adult
Rating: Fair
Format of test: The child is asked to follow commands, answer questions, fill in missing words, read a story and answer questions about it, and write sentences and paragraphs.

38. Lindamood Auditory Conceptualization Test (Lindamood & Lindamood, 1971)
Areas tested (speech and language): Comprehension
Areas tested (processing): Discrimination and perception of speech sounds
For ages: Kindergarten to 12th grade
Rating: Poor
Format of test: The child is given various colored blocks and told that they represent different sounds. The task is to "spell" various words with the blocks.

39. Michigan Picture Language Inventory (Lerea & Wolski, 1962)
Areas tested (speech and language): Comprehension and expression
For ages: 4–6 years
Rating: Fair
Format of test: Sentences are presented with missing words. The child must say the missing word and must point to the correct pictures in a book.

40. Northwestern Syntax Screening Test (NSST) (Lee, 1971)
Areas tested (speech and language): Expressive and receptive language
For ages: 3–8 years
Rating: Fair
Format of test: Two subtests: (1) Child must select picture that

represents stimulus sentence read by examiner, and (2) child must repeat stimulus sentences.

41. Oral Language Sentence Imitation Test (OLSIT) (Zachman, Huisingh, Jorgensen, & Barrett, 1977)
Areas tested (speech and language): Expressive language
Areas tested (processing): Sentence imitation
For ages: Not normed
Rating: Fair
Format of test: The child must repeat sentences of differing levels of grammatical complexity.
42. Peabody Picture Vocabulary Test (PPVT) (Dunn & Dunn, 1981)
Areas tested (speech and language): Receptive vocabulary
For ages: 2 years through adult
Rating: Good
Format of test: Child must point to picture that represents stimulus word.
43. Photo Articulation Test (Pendergast, Dickey, Selmar, & Soder, 1969)
Areas tested (speech and language): Speech articulation
For ages: 3 through 12 years
Rating: Fair
Format of test: Naming
44. Picture Articulation and Language Screening Test (Rodgers, 1976)
Areas tested (speech and language): Speech articulation
For ages: Not normed
Rating: Fair
Format of test: Naming
45. Porch Index of Communicative Ability in Children (PICAC) (Porch, 1975)
Areas tested (speech and language): Verbal, gestural, and written comprehension and expression of concepts
Areas tested (processing): Visual matching, verbal imitation (words)
For ages: Not normed at present; geared for ages 3–12 years
Rating: Fair
Format of test: A variety of subtests, including naming objects; showing functions of objects; supplying missing words in sentences; following auditory commands; matching pictures and objects; and reading and writing words.
46. Preschool Language Assessment Instrument (Blank, Rose, & Berlin, 1978)
Areas tested (speech and language): Language expression and comprehension

For ages: 3–6 years
Rating: Fair
Format of test: The child must follow commands and respond to questions.

47. Preschool Language Scale (Zimmerman, Steiner, & Evatt, 1969)
Areas tested: Comprehension and expression
For ages: 18 months to 7 years
Rating: Fair to poor
Format of test: There are two parts to this test: comprehension, where the child must point to vocabulary items; and expression, where the child must repeat sentences, name objects, and form sentences.

48. Receptive–Expressive–Emergent Language Scale (Bzoch & League, 1970)
Areas tested (speech and language): Expressive and receptive language
For ages: 1–3 years
Rating: Fair
Format of test: Scale of behaviors depends upon maternal interview responses.

49. Riley Articulation and Language Test (RALT) (Riley, 1971)
Areas tested (speech and language): Speech articulation
For ages: Kindergarten to second grade
Rating: Fair
Format of test: Naming

50. Roswell–Chall Auditory Blending Test (Roswell & Chall, 1963)
Areas tested (processing): Sound blending
For ages: First to fourth grades
Rating: Fair
Format of test: The examiner says words, at the rate of ½ second per sound. The child must say the word at a normal rate.

51. Screening Test for Auditory Perception (Kimmell & Wahl, 1969)
Areas tested (processing): Auditory discrimination and memory for sounds and sequences
For ages: Second through sixth grades
Rating: Poor
Format of test: There are a variety of subtests, including determining if pairs of words are "same" or "different"; reproducing series of tapped rhythms; and picking out rhyming words from strings of words. The instructions for the various subtests are rather difficult.

52. Screening Test of Adolescent Language (STAL) (Prather, Breecher, Stafford, & Wallace, 1980)
Areas tested: Expressive and receptive language

For ages: Sixth through ninth grade
Rating: Fair to good
Format of test: Four subtests in which the child must (1) give synonyms ("vocabulary"); (2) repeat sentences ("auditory memory span"); (3) state whether sentences are correct or nonsense ("language processing"); and (4) paraphrase proverbs read by the examiner ("proverb explanation").

53. Sequenced Inventory of Communication Development (Hedrick, Prather, & Tobin, 1975)
Areas tested (speech and language): Expressive and receptive language
Areas tested (processing): Discrimination of environmental sounds; auditory memory
For ages: 4 months to 4 years
Rating: Fair
Format of test: The test is composed of over 200 items, with tasks including imitating words and sounds; responding to questions; and carrying out commands with toys.
54. Short Term Auditory Retrieval and Storage (Flowers, 1972)
Areas tested (processing): Auditory discrimination and memory for words
For ages: First to sixth grades
Rating: Poor
Format of test: Child is presented with two stimulus words simultaneously (on tape), and must select picture in answer book that represents the two words.
55. *Sound Discrimination Test* (Templin, 1956)
Areas tested (processing): Auditory discrimination of speech sounds
For ages: Not normed; geared for "school age"
Rating: Fair to poor
Format of test: The child is presented with pairs of nonsense words and asked to determine if they are the same or different.
56. Southwestern Spanish Articulation Test (Toronto, 1977a)
Areas tested (speech and language): Speech articulation
For ages: Not normed
Rating: Fair to good
Format of test: Naming in Spanish
57. Templin–Darley Tests of Articulation (Templin & Darley, 1969)
Areas tested (speech and language): Speech articulation
For ages: 3 through 8 years
Rating: Fair to good
Format of test: Naming pictures
58. Test of Auditory Comprehension of Language (TACL) (Carrow, 1978)

Areas tested (speech and language): Receptive language (English or Spanish)
For ages: 3–7 years
Rating: Good
Format of test: Child must select picture that represents stimulus item read by examiner. Stimuli include vocabulary items, grammatical elements, and sentence structures.

59. Test of Adolescent Language (TOAL) (Hammill, Brown, Larsen, & Wiederholt, 1980)
Areas tested (speech and language): Receptive and expressive language
Areas tested (processing): Memory for sentences, reading, and writing
For ages: 11–17.5 years
Rating: Fair
Format of test: The test consists of eight subtests, including (1) selecting two pictures representing two aspects of the meaning of a stimulus word; (2) selecting which two of three sentences have the same meaning with sentences presented orally and in writing; (3) forming sentences using a stimulus word; (4) repeating sentences; and (5) selecting words that "go together" semantically.

60. Test of Concept Utilization (TCU) (Crager, 1972)
Areas tested (speech and language): Expressive language
For ages: 1st through 12 grade
Rating: Fair
Format of test: The child is presented with stimulus words and must explain how they are alike.

61. Test of Early Language Development (TELD) (Hresko, Reid, & Hammill, 1981)
Areas tested (speech and language): Receptive and expressive language
For ages: 3.0–7.11 years
Rating: Fair to good
Format of test: Child must point to pictures representing stimulus words and sentences, and must answer questions.

62. Test of Language Development (TOLD) (Newcomer & Hammill, 1977)
Areas tested (speech and language): Receptive and expressive language
Areas tested (processing): Auditory memory (sentences) and discrimination
For ages: 4–9 years
Rating: Good
Format of test: Various subtests, in which the child must point to stimulus items ("grammatic understanding," "picture vocabu-

lary"); define words ("oral vocabulary"); repeat sentences ("sentence imitation"); complete sentences with missing words ("grammatic completion"); and state whether pairs of words are "same" or "different" ("word discrimination").

63. Token Test for Children (DiSimoni, 1978)
Areas tested (speech and language): Receptive language
Areas tested (processing): Auditory memory (sentences)
For ages: 3–12 years
Rating: Good
Format of test: The child must carry out commands of differing length and complexity.

64. Toronto Tests of Receptive Vocabulary English/Spanish (TTRV) (Toronto, 1977b)
Areas tested (speech and language): Receptive vocabulary, English and Spanish
For ages: 4–10 years
Rating: Fair
Format of test: The child must point to the pictures in a book that best represent the stimuli read to him by the examiner.

65. Utah Test of Language Development (Mecham, Jex, & Jones, 1967)
Areas tested (speech and language): Receptive and expressive skills (overall measure)
For ages: 18 months to 14.5 years
Rating: Fair to poor
Format of test: Child must point out body parts, follow simple commands, name vocabulary items, repeat digits, read, and write.

66. Verbal Language Development Scale (Mecham, 1958)
Areas tested (speech and language): General measure
For ages: 1–14 years
Rating: Poor
Format of test: Language scale is completed using interview responses from the mother or other informant.

67. Visual Aural Digit Span Test (VADS) (Koppitz, 1977)
Areas tested (processing): Auditory and visual memory for digits
For ages: 5.6–12.11 years
Rating: Fair
Format of test: Combinations of aural versus visual presentation and aural versus visual recall for digit strings.

68. Vocabulary Comprehension Scale (T. E. Bangs, 1975)
Areas tested (speech and language): Language comprehension
For ages: Not normed; aimed at ages 2–6 years

Rating: Fair
Format of test: The child must point to, or follow commands with, a set of toy objects.

69. Wechsler Intelligence Scale for Children—Revised (WISC-R) (Wechsler, 1974)
Areas tested (processing): Nonverbal intelligence, verbal intelligence, and "full-scale" intelligence
For ages: 6–17 years
Rating: Good
Format of test: The nonverbal part of the test consists of identifying missing parts of pictures; arranging pictures in logical sequential order; constructing designs with blocks; assembling puzzles; and associating signs and symbols. The verbal part of the test consists of answering information and "comprehension" questions; stating how two words are similar; solving arithmetic problems; and completing analogies. Supplementary subtests include mazes and forward and backward digit span.

70. Wechsler Preschool and Primary Scale or Intelligence (WPPSI) (Wechsler, 1967)
Areas tested (processing): Nonverbal intelligence, verbal intelligence, and "full-scale" intelligence
For ages: 4–6.5 years
Rating: Fair (verbal subtests) to good (nonverbal tests)
Format of test: The nonverbal part of the test consists of constructing designs with blocks; associating signs and symbols; identifying missing parts of pictures; solving mazes; and copying designs. The verbal part of the test consists of answering information questions; defining vocabulary items; solving arithmetic problems; completing analogies; and imitating sentences.

CHAPTER 4

Differential Diagnosis of Syndromes Involving Disorders of Speech and Language Development

Introduction

Once it has been determined that a child has some abnormal speech or language development, the question of differential diagnosis arises. There are a number of syndromes that involve abnormal speech or language development as one of their presenting features. In this chapter, detailed descriptions are given of the clinical features found in the syndromes of developmental language disorder and developmental articulation disorder. In addition, descriptions are given of the clinical features found in other childhood syndromes that involve language or speech disorders and are relevant to the differential diagnosis of either developmental language disorder or developmental articulation disorder. The other syndromes included are acquired childhood language disorder ("aphasia"), hearing impairment, mental retardation, elective mutism, organic disorders involving articulation, and childhood psychoses (including the schizophrenias, infantile autism, and pervasive developmental disorder). Following the clinical descriptions of the various syndromes, a summary chart for making differential diagnoses is presented, and an outline is provided as to how to go about establishing a differential diagnosis.

We wish to preface our discussion of syndromes involving abnormal language development with the disclaimer that, while these categories may delineate separate psychiatric diagnostic categories, it is not yet clear that each of these categories represents a unique type of linguistic disorder. In addition, there is often overlap between or among these psychiatric syndromes. For example, the majority of children with infantile autism also have some degree of mental retardation. A "rubella child" frequently has both mental retardation and hearing impairment, and may show autistic-like behavioral syndromes as well.

Developmental Language Disorder

The features of developmental language disorder vary, depending upon the severity of the disorder and the age of the child affected. In general, however, nonlinguistic functioning (including hearing acuity, intellectual functioning, neurological functioning, "inner language," behavior, and communicative intent) is grossly normal. Although minor abnormalities may be present in nonlinguistic areas, these are not sufficiently severe to account for the lack of normal language development found in the child.

Nonlinguistic Features

In children with developmental language disorder, hearing levels are usually within normal limits. If these children do suffer hearing loss, the auditory impairment is insufficient to account for the language deficit. Nonetheless, in younger children, and in children with more severe forms of developmental language disorder, there is often the clinical impression of significant hearing loss. A history of inconsistent auditory responses, partial hearing impairment, recurrent otitis media, or even ambiguous audiograms may be present.

Aside from a history of recurrent otitis media, the medical history of the child with developmental language disorder is usually normal. A small number of children with developmental language disorder may show neurological "soft signs" (DeHirsch, 1975).

Intellectual functioning (except for verbal areas) is usually within normal limits, and may even be in the superior range. In cases where nonverbal intelligence is impaired, it is not impaired to a sufficient degree to account for the language deficit. Among younger children with developmental language disorder, careful testing is often necessary, since the children's inability to understand instructions may give the incorrect impression of intellectual deficits.

"Inner language" is present in children with developmental language disorder, and is evidenced in even quite young children by appropriate use of toys and objects and in older children by imaginative or creative patterns of play. The make-believe play of a child with developmental language disorder may be somewhat less complex than is usual for the child's age level.

While developmental and motor skills are usually within normal limits in children with developmental language disorder, a history of delay in reaching some motor or developmental milestones is not uncommon. Motor coordination impairments seem to be the most commonly associated developmental disorders found in these children, although enuresis and encopresis do occur at somewhat higher rates than would be expected in the general population.

Among school-age children, learning disorders, particularly specific developmental reading disorder and mixed developmental learning disorder, are extremely common. Various specific cognitive skills (usually involving auditory processing, but sometimes affecting visual processing) may show some impairment. Again, careful testing is required, since the nature of learning problems in these children may be obscured by multiple and serious behavioral problems in the classroom.

Behavioral and emotional problems are common associated features in children with developmental language disorder. Those children whose receptive language skills are affected are more likely to have such problems than are children with purely expressive involvement. Among the more common behavioral and emotional problems are attentional deficits and anxiety disorders. (A more detailed discussion of the behavioral and emotional problems of these children is provided in Chapter 6.)

Despite emotional and behavioral problems, children with developmental language disorder usually appear friendly and show a desire to communicate. Even quite young children evidence this by maintaining eye contact, relating well with the mother, and enjoying games such as pat-a-cake and peek-a-boo. In older children with developmental language disorder, the desire to communicate is manifested by the use of vocalizations, gestures, and eye contact. In extreme cases of receptive impairment, however, there may be some depression of these features.

Linguistic Features

The language of children with developmental language disorder typically shows abnormalities in almost all areas, although the types of abnormalities and the extent of the abnormalities vary from case to case. Younger children tend to show more global problems, with articulation, vocabulary, grammar, and the contextual use of language all showing some disturbances, while older children may have "outgrown" problems in certain areas (articulation is one of the first areas to recover) and may only show problems in isolated aspects of language.

Although some research has attempted to delineate subtypes of developmental language disorder, the question of subtypes is still being debated. It is clear that there are at least two major subtypes of the disorder: a purely expressive one, in which comprehension skills are not affected, and a receptive one, in which both expressive and comprehension skills are affected. These two major subtypes are recognized in DSM-III as well as by a large number of authors (Crookes & Greene,

1963; DeHirsch, 1975; Eisenson, 1972; N. Gordon, 1966; McGinnis, 1963; Myklebust, 1983), although the terminology for the two subtypes has differed with different authors. Among the more common terms for the expressive subtype are "expressive aphasia," "motor aphasia," "mild developmental language disorder," and "Broca's aphasia." Among the more common terms for the receptive subtype are "receptive aphasia," "sensory aphasia," "Wernicke's aphasia," "moderate developmental language disorder," and "severe developmental language disorder." More recent research has led a number of authors to define a larger number of subtypes of developmental language disorder (Aram & Nation, 1975; Chappell, 1970; Richman & Lindgren, 1980; Wolfus, Moscovitch, & Kinsbourne, 1980). Since precise definitions of subgroups of impairments in children with developmental language disorder are not agreed upon beyond the major divisions of receptive versus purely expressive impairment, the present discussion refers only to these two broad subtypes.

The speech of children with developmental language disorder virtually always shows some disturbances at some point in time. Typically, the articulation of speech sounds (particularly consonants) is less accurate than in normal children of the same age; the overall intelligibility of speech is decreased; and there may be associated dysfluency or stuttering.

The articulation abnormalities of children with developmental language disorder include omissions, distortions, or substitutions of consonant sounds. However, nonarticulatory oral motor functions, such as chewing and swallowing, are typically normal. The articulation of speech may be somewhat variable in children with developmental language disorder, with certain sounds being correctly articulated at some times and incorrectly articulated at other times. In addition, the children may have difficulties with the ordering of speech sounds within words.

The speech dysfluencies of children with developmental language disorder are usually transient, and do not occur in all cases. When present, the speech dysfluencies consist of repetitions or interjections of which the child is not aware. The significance and the cause of these speech dysfluencies is not known. Some researchers have suggested that these dysfluencies are manifestations of word-finding difficulties, and other researchers have suggested that the dysfluencies may be the result of the "stress" of speech therapy.

The intonation patterns of the speech of children with developmental language disorder are usually normal.

Vocabulary is one area of language development that can show a wide range of involvement in developmental language disorder, from almost normal (with only very subtle disturbances involving only certain types of words) to widely disturbed. In general, however, the vocabulary of children with developmental language disorder is limited (in terms of both the number of words known and the frequency with which different words are used) in comparison to children of the same age without developmental language disorder. In addition, children with developmental language disorder typically have marked difficulty learning new words, and may require as many as 30 examples before they can come to understand a new word.

Vocabulary comprehension deficits tend to be widespread in younger children with developmental language disorder. Older children with developmental language disorder, however, often score within normal limits on global tests of vocabulary such as the PPVT (German, 1979). In older children with developmental language disorder, vocabulary comprehension deficits tend to be limited to certain types of words, such as spatial, temporal, or kinship terms (Wiig & Semel, 1973).

Vocabulary expression deficits may affect all types of words and may be manifested in a variety of ways. For example, the child may use substitutions ("table" for "chair"), functional descriptions ("sit on" for "chair"), overgeneralizations ("thing" for "chair"), or jargon ("pabim" for "chair") instead of the correct word, or the child may produce the correct word, but only after long hesitations, "ums," and "ers." In older children with less severe forms of developmental language disorder, vocabulary expression deficits may be limited to words involving abstract concepts (such as "democracy").

The course of language development in children with developmental language disorder is slower than normal, with the children typically beginning to speak later and advancing to each stage of language development very slowly. The amount of time such children spend in each stage of language development varies widely from child to child, but may be as much as several years at a given stage. Furthermore, the rate of language development in children with developmental language disorder is typically uneven from stage to stage. The stages of language development may also be less clear-cut than in normal children. For example, one-word utterances may remain after a child can form sentences.

The course of language acquisition in these children is controversial. It is still open to question whether children with developmental language disorder are simply "delayed" (i.e., they follow the normal course of stages of language development, but at a slower rate than is usual), or whether they are "deviant" in their patterns of language acquisition (Lee, 1966; Leonard, 1972; Menyuk, 1964; Morehead & Ingram, 1973).

The grammatical structures produced by children with developmental language disorder are typically simplified in comparison to those produced by normal children of the same age. The simplifications found include shorter sentences, limited varieties of sentence structures, and omissions of certain types of words or structures (e.g., prepositions, indefinite pronouns, verbal auxiliaries, conjunctions, negatives, or verbal endings) (Leonard, 1972). In addition to producing sentences with grammatical errors, children with developmental language disorder are often unable to recognize deviant sentences when produced by others (Liles, Shulman & Bartlett, 1977).

Sometimes the grammatical structures produced by children with developmental language disorder are grossly abnormal, consisting only of strings of nouns ("Mommy car, dog car") or of unusual word orders ("car Mommy have"). But more frequently, the differences in the grammar of children with developmental language disorder are quantitative rather than qualitative; the actual forms generated are similar to those generated by normal children, but the variety in forms is less common (Johnston & Schery, 1976; Morehead & Ingram, 1973). In older children with developmental language disorder, grammatical problems may be limited to "higher-level" (later-learned) sentence constructions, involving subject + adjective versus object + adjective constructions (Bryen & Gerber, 1981).

As stated above, the language comprehension of children

with developmental language disorder may be age-appropriate or severely limited. Often comprehension is partially limited, with the child able to follow simple commands but unable to follow more complex ones. Auditory memory may also play a role in the comprehension abilities of children with developmental language disorder; these children have been shown to have increased comprehension difficulties as a function of increased utterance length (Aram & Nation, 1982).

The auditory processing of children with developmental language disorder may be abnormal in a variety of areas, including auditory discrimination, auditory memory, and auditory–visual integration. (This is discussed in greater detail in Chapter 2.)

The ways in which children with developmental language disorder use language may also be abnormal to some degree. The verbal responses of these children, particularly in the younger years, may be somewhat "off target" or may consist largely of echolalia. Self-corrections of linguistic errors by these children are extremely rare. In severe cases, responses may be tangential, perseverative, or completely inappropriate. Even in older children with fairly well-developed language systems, there tend to be difficulties in understanding the more subtle aspects of conversations, resulting in occasional inappropriate responses. Studies have shown that such children tend to be less assertive conversational partners than normal children and seem to be unable to understand the significance of "politeness" forms (Bryan, Donahue, & Pearl, 1981; Donahue, 1981).

Further discussion of the clinical features of developmental language disorder may be found in Chapter 5.

Developmental Articulation Disorder

Nonlinguistic Features

Developmental articulation disorder is essentially a disorder of speech articulation. Intelligence level, hearing acuity, and speech mechanism structures are not affected, and other nonlinguistic and linguistic areas of functioning are generally within normal limits.

The features sometimes associated with developmental articulation disorder include developmental problems, social or emotional problems, behavioral problems, and neurological problems. The most commonly reported developmental problems are enuresis, developmental coordination disorder, and learning disabilities, which, together, affect about 25% of the children with developmental articulation disorder. A larger proportion of these children have slow early speech or language milestones. Although it is a reasonable assumption that reading and spelling difficulties in these children affect the same sounds that are misarticulated, research has not shown an association between misarticulations and reading or spelling errors.

While no clear associations between neurological disorders and developmental articulation disorder have been found, children with developmental articulation disorder have been shown as a group to have slightly elevated incidences of neurological "soft signs," especially clumsiness and mixed dominance. Case history reports frequently mention left–right confusions in these children, although there are no systematic studies on this topic.

Case reports also suggest that children with developmental articulation disorder have a high prevalence of social, emotional, or behavioral problems. Our research (discussed in Chapter 6) shows that approximately one-third of these children have some diagnosable psychiatric disorder. Children with severe or persistent impairments appear to be the ones most likely to suffer from psychiatric problems. The most common psychiatric problems in these children are anxieties, peer problems, poor self-images, and attention or concentration deficits.

Linguistic Features

The essential feature of developmental articulation disorder is articulation that is judged to be defective when compared to speakers of the same dialect at the same age level, and that is not due to abnormalities in intelligence, hearing, or physiology of the speech mechanism.

Although there is some controversy as to the presence of

subtle deficits in language development among children with developmental articulation disorder (see Chapter 2 for a more detailed discussion), it appears that these children's understanding of language, use of language to communicate, and ability to form sentences and express concepts is within normal limits.

The misarticulations made by children with developmental articulation disorder are of three different types: omissions of speech sounds, distortions of speech sounds, or substitutions of one speech sound for another. The sounds that are most frequently misarticulated in this disorder are those that tend to be acquired last in the normal language acquisition process. These include /s/, /z/, /sh/, /ch/, /dg/, /dz/, /th/, (as in "thumb"), /dh/ (as in "these"), and /r/. In severe cases involving younger children, some of the earlier-learned phonemes may be affected (e.g., /b/, /m/, /t/, /d/, /n/, and /h/). Misarticulations of vowel sounds are not usually found in this disorder. Misarticulations tend to occur most frequently in the middle or ends of words. Although the misarticulations tend to affect the more "difficult" (i.e., the later-acquired) speech sounds, it is important to keep in mind that these children's misarticulations reflect an inadequate or deviant phonological system rather than an inability to execute certain articulatory movements (Pollack & Rees, 1972).

The most frequently occurring type of misarticulation is the substitution of one phoneme or speech sound for another. Among the more frequently found substitutions are /th/ for /s/ ("thithorth" for "scissors"), /w/ for /r/ ("wabbit" for "rabbit"), /b/ for /v/ ("shobel" for "shovel"), /f/ for /th/ ("fum" for "thumb"), /p/ for /f/ ("leap" for "leaf"), /d/ for /dh/ ("dis" for "this"), /w/ for /l/ ("wook" for "look"), and /y/ for /l/ ("Yeyo" for "yellow") (Snow, 1963). In general, substitutions are made between sounds that are of similar types: Voiced sounds tend to be substituted for voiced sounds, voiceless sounds for voiceless sounds, labial sounds for labial sounds, and so on. As noted above, substitution errors tend to be found more frequently when the sound occurs in the middle or end of a word than when it occurs at the beginning of a word.

The second most common type of misarticulation is the omission of a phoneme. Omissions are most frequently found in the speech of younger children and usually occur at the ends of words or in clusters of consonants. Some typical examples of the omission found in the speech of children with developmental articulation disorder are "ka" for "car," "ow" for "house," "scisso" for "scissors," "kitma" for "Christmas," and "bu" for "blue."

The third type of misarticulation found in the speech of children with developmental articulation disorder is distortion or misarticulation resulting in a sound that is not part of the dialect. Distortions are found mainly in older children and may be the last type of misarticulation remaining in the speech of children whose misarticulations have mostly remitted. The most common types of distortions found are the lateral lisp (in which the child pronounces /s/ sounds with the air stream going across the tongue, producing a whistle-like effect) and the palatal lisp (in which the /s/ sound is formed with the tongue too close to the palate, producing a "shh"-like effect).

There is a considerable range in the severity of developmental articulation disorder. Since misarticulations may affect from one to many sounds and may be of one or more types, the effect of these misarticulations on communication can range from miniscule to extreme. A child with developmental articulation disorder may produce speech that is 100% intelligible (e.g., a child who only omits the phoneme /r/ at the ends of words) or speech that is only partially intelligible. It is easy to see how a child whose articulation problems include a variety of types of errors and a variety of affected phonemes could produce speech that is completely unintelligible. Indeed, several studies have shown that children with severe forms of developmental articulation disorder produce speech that is so deviant that the children themselves are unable to decode samples of their own speech.

The misarticulations of children with developmental articulation disorder are often described as "inconsistent." It appears that the misarticulations of these children are random; a child may pronounce a phoneme correctly one time and incorrectly another time. However, there are actually a number of factors governing the correct or incorrect articulation of speech sounds in these children, and there is usually a certain amount of consistency among the misarticulations. Among the factors that condition the presence of misarticulations are these: the position in the word where the sound occurs (misarticulations, as noted, are more frequent at the ends of words; type of utterance (misarticulations are more frequent in long, syntactically complex sentences than in short sentences or single-word utterances); type of word (misarticulations are more common in simpler, earlier-learned words); and type of speech (misarticulations are more common during rapid speech).

As is the case with developmental language disorder, there is controversy as to whether developmental articulation disorder involves essentially "delayed" or "deviant" articulation. Many of the processes of simplifying adult forms of speech that are found in the speech of children with developmental articulation disorder are present in the speech of younger normal children. Such processes include reducing consonant clusters ("bu" for "blue"), reduplicating consonant clusters ("baba" for "bottle"), substituting stop sounds for fricative sounds ("pat" for "fat"), and substituting glides for /r/ ("wed" for "red"). It appears that these processes persist longer in the speech of children with developmental articulation disorder than they do in the speech of normal children (Ingram, 1976; R. Schwartz, Leonard, Folger, & Wilcox, 1980).

In addition, it appears that certain children with developmental articulation disorder use unique processes not found in the speech of normal children. These processes include substitution of /t/ for /f/, /m/ for /w/, and voiced sounds for voiceless ones preceding vowels (Hodson & Paden, 1981; Ingram, 1976; Leonard, 1973; Pollack & Rees, 1972). The presence of such abnormal processes has not, however, been documented in all children with developmental articulation disorder (R. Schwartz *et al.*, 1980).

Various studies have suggested that there is a "sound preference" among some children with developmental articulation disorder. Ingram (1976) describes some children who preferred nasal or fricative sounds over others, and F. Weiner (1981) describes children who preferred the /h/ sound in their substitutions.

Acquired Childhood Language Disorder ("Aphasia")

Instances of "true aphasia" (loss of acquired language as a result of cerebral trauma) are rare in children. The literature, which consists of a limited number of case reports, indicates that there are two types of circumstances in which children manifest what appears to be an acquired (rather than a developmental) language disorder. In the first circumstance there is known cerebral trauma (usually the result of auto accidents, but sometimes the result of brain pathology). In the second there is a progressive loss of acquired language concomitant with the appearance of a convulsive disorder.

Acquired Childhood Language Disorder with Cerebral Trauma

The effects of cerebral trauma in childhood are apparently dependent upon both the extent of the damage and the age at which the damage occurs. The literature suggests that the effects are less marked in cases of unilateral lesions in early childhood (before the age of 7 years) and more severe in cases of bilateral lesions in young children or unilateral (left) lesions in older children.

NONLINGUISTIC FEATURES

Because acquired childhood aphasia can result from several different types of cerebral injuries, a variety of other, nonlinguistic features may be found. The most common of these are right hemiplegias or less global motor impairments involving the right side of the body.

LINGUISTIC FEATURES

Early reports have suggested that the linguistic effects of unilateral lesions in young children are completely transient, and it has been hypothesized that this is because of the plasticity of the young brain, which results in a transfer of brain functions from the damaged hemisphere to the undamaged hemisphere (Alajouanine & Lhermitte, 1965; Lenneberg, 1967). Later reports, however, have shown that, while children with these unilateral lesions early in life do tend to develop language eventually, they may in fact have some type of lasting linguistic impairments (Hecaen, 1976; Woods & Carey, 1979). It appears that for children whose brain trauma occurs after the age of 7 years, some recovery from the initial language loss will occur, but the likelihood of lasting and significant linguistic impairments is high (Hagen, 1981; Oelschlaeger & Scarborough, 1976).

Because of the limited data available on children with acquired aphasia, little is known about the types of linguistic impairments found. The linguistic feature that most authors report finding in children with acquired aphasia (and that seems to be a major difference between the acquired aphasia of children and the acquired aphasia of adults) is a marked decrease in the use of all expressive language, which has been labeled "hypoproductivity" (Guttman, 1942). Many of these children simply stop talking altogether for a period of time ranging from several weeks to years (Hecaen, 1976). Following the return of speech, these children show severe verbal inhibition and must be prompted and prodded to produce verbal responses. Disorders of language comprehension are less frequent and of shorter duration in acquired childhood aphasia than are disorders involving expression.

The other initial linguistic disturbances that have been reported in children with acquired aphasia of this type are dysarthrias, speech hesitations, and telegraphic utterances (Guttman, 1942); expressive language disorder characterized by severe perseveration and impairment of graphemic skills (Wanderley & Lefevre, 1969); varying degrees of articulation impairment, expressive grammatical impairments, comprehension disorders, and naming difficulties (Hecaen, 1976); deficits in picture naming, completing sentences, answering relational questions, and following commands (Woods & Carey, 1979); complete lack of comprehension and expressive abilities; and an inability to read or to copy written words (Oelschlaeger & Scarborough, 1976).

Apparently, during the period of recovery from acquired childhood aphasia, the course of language development that occurs does not follow normal patterns. Lenneberg (1967) describes aphasia in a young child as a few weeks or months of unresponsiveness, followed by language acquisition at a faster than normal rate. A more detailed description (Yeni-Komshian, 1977) reports that the recovery of articulation abilities occurs at a faster rate than the recovery of naming abilities.

Oelschlaeger and Scarborough (1976) report a case where understanding of language and ability to respond to simple questions returned, but ability to form grammatical sentences remained disturbed. Woods and Carey (1979) describe a group of seven recovered childhood aphasics who showed significant impairments in picture naming, spelling, clause formation, and sentence completion tasks.

Acquired Childhood Language Disorder with Associated Convulsive Disorder

A large number of case reports describe a sudden and progressive loss of language functions in children, associated with an abnormal EEG and usually with convulsive disorder (Deonna, Beaumanior, Gaillard, & Assal, 1977).

NONLINGUISTIC FEATURES

The developmental and medical histories of these children are apparently unremarkable prior to the onset of the disorder, which can occur anywhere between the ages of 3 and 13 years, but is usually between the ages of 4 and 7 years. Family history is usually negative for speech, language, and seizure disorders. Onset is not associated with trauma or with acute illness, although there have been case reports of some children having onset following otitis media (Shoumaker, Bennett, Bray, & Curless, 1974). Etiology of the disorder is unknown, although the fluctuating course of recovery has caused some authors to postulate an underlying inflammatory process (McKinney & McGreal, 1974). A number of authors hypothesize that a slow viral infection is involved (Gascon, Victor, Lombroso, & Goodglass, 1973; Lou, Brandt, & Bruhn, 1977; Shoumaker *et al.*, 1974). Nonetheless, laboratory findings are normal on cerebrospinal fluid examinations, pneumoencephalograms, and angiograms.

The most striking nonlinguistic feature of this type of acquired childhood language disorder is the onset of seizure activity and/or EEG abnormalities. EEG disturbances are usually bilateral, but, if unilateral, are not necessarily on the dominant side according to handedness. Reports suggest that EEG abnormalities are usually more prominent in the temporal lobe region, but may be widespread. The seizures are generally responsive to anticonvulsant treatment.

There are apparently no major effects on general development (Deonna, Fletcher, & Voumard, 1982), on neurological status, or on nonverbal intelligence levels. A literature review shows that over 85% of the children with this disorder have normal nonverbal intelligence levels (Miller, Campbell, Champa, & Weismer, 1984). However, there have been some isolated case reports of visual–perceptual impairments (Mantovani & Landau, 1980) and neurological dysfunctions (Van-Dongen & Loonen, 1977).

Various behavioral and emotional problems have been reported in these children, including withdrawal, inattention, tantrums, and hyperactivity. These problems apparently occur with the onset of the disorder and frequently disappear once an alternative communication system is established (Campbell & Heaton, 1978).

LINGUISTIC FEATURES

The types of linguistic dysfunctions found in acquired childhood language disorder with associated convulsive disorder have not been well described in the literature, and the only generalization that can be made at present is that both receptive and expressive language appear to be affected.

Onset and course of the linguistic disorder vary considerably. Some authors have reported that linguistic deficits are slow in developing and may be mistaken for psychological problems (Humphrey, Knipstein, & Bumpass, 1975); others report an abrupt loss of language comprehension and failure to respond to sounds, giving the impression of sudden deafness (Worster-Drought, 1971). However, in cases of children who suddenly appear deaf, their hearing levels (as assessed by audiograms) are usually normal. Although there are no epidemiological data, it appears that the majority of cases present with an abrupt onset.

Recovery among reported cases is also variable; some children show a steady progressive recovery of language abilities over time, while others show marked fluctuations in all areas of language abilities over time. A literature review (Miller *et al.*, 1984) indicates that in 94% of cases problems persist or recur beyond 6 months after onset. While both language and EEGs do improve over time, it is unclear whether the improvement in language skills parallels the improvement in EEGs.

The language comprehension disorder involved in this syndrome is pervasive and seems to be the first language disturbance to appear (L. Jordan, 1980; Watters, 1974). The severity of the comprehension disorder is apparent in case reports that describe the patient as having "the appearance of being deaf," as well as in the report (Landau & Kleffner, 1957) of a 15-year-old boy who returned to normal, but who stated that during the disorder he perceived speech as "blah, blah, blah." In children who have acquired reading ability prior to the onset of the disorder, their comprehension of written material, as well as of spoken material, is found to be disrupted with the disorder.

In addition to comprehension difficulties, disorders in auditory discrimination and auditory processing have been reported (Campbell & Heaton, 1978; L. Jordan, 1980).

Speech is also affected. Some children become totally mute, and others vocalize only by grunts. Unusual articulation errors, such as additions of sounds or syllables in words (e.g., "crouge" for "rouge"), have been reported (Deonna *et al.*, 1982); these occur in addition to the more usual types of articulation errors involving substitutions, distortions, or omissions of sounds. In some children, abnormalities in voice quality have been reported along with abnormal patterns of intonation (Cooper & Ferry, 1978; Worster-Drought, 1971).

Case reports suggest that virtually all areas of expressive language development may be affected: word fluency, object-naming skills, and quantity of expressive language (in terms of both number of utterances and length of utterances).

Hearing Impairment

Like the term "developmental language disorder," the term "hearing impairment" covers a wide range of disorders—from the minor transient difficulties in perceiving certain speech sounds that might result from an ear infection, to the quite devastating condition of deafness in which speech cannot be understood at all. The different degrees of hearing impairment are usually defined in terms of thresholds of sensitivity to pure tones in the frequencies used for speech (500, 1000, and 2000 Hz). The American Academy of Ophthalmology and Otolaryngology has presented a classification relating the degree of hearing thresholds to the difficulty in understanding speech (H. Davis & Kranz, 1964; Silverman, 1971). This classification suggests that hearing thresholds of 40 dB or less produce difficulty only with faint speech; hearing thresholds of more than 40 dB produce difficulty with normal speech.

The type of hearing loss is also significant for the understanding of speech (Northern & Downs, 1978). Certain types of hearing loss may affect only sounds having frequencies above 200 Hz (high-frequency hearing loss). Individuals with such hearing loss will have difficulty understanding words with the /f/, /s/, or /th/ sounds in them. Individuals with hearing loss confined to frequencies above 1000 Hz will have difficulty recognizing words with /p/, /g/, /ch/, or /sh/ sounds as well.

Nonlinguistic Features

Assessment of intelligence in children with hearing loss is difficult, because of the verbal nature of most intelligence tests. However, when this complicating factor is controlled for, the intelligence levels of most hearing-impaired children usually fall in the normal range (Bonvillian, Nelson, & Charrow, 1973; J. Wilson, Rapin, Wilson, & VanDenburg, 1975). Various early studies have shown that the way in which children with severe or profound hearing loss acquire knowledge about the world is the same as, or only slightly delayed in comparison with, that of normal children (H. G. Furth, 1961; H. L. Furth, 1971). However, a certain number of children with severe or profound hearing loss do show associated mental retardation. This is most likely to occur in cases where hearing loss has been caused by head trauma, meningitis, or maternal rubella.

Similarly, medical problems are commonly found in some children with hearing loss. The medical factors determined by the American Association of Otolaryngology as being high-risk factors for hearing loss are (1) history of familial hereditary deafness; (2) maternal rubella; (3) fetal infections; (4) defects of the nose, ear, or throat; (5) birth weight of less than 1500 grams; (6) bilirubin levels of more than 20 milligrams per 100 milliliters of serum; and (7) congenital cytomegalovirus (Lloyd & Dahle, 1976).

Play tends to be normal in children with hearing loss, and such children use toys and objects appropriately.

A significantly high prevalence of visual abnormalities (including defects in acuity, fusion, and color vision) has also been found in children with hearing loss (J. Wilson *et al.*, 1975).

A higher frequency of behavioral and emotional problems has been reported in hearing-impaired than in normal children. The most prevalent problems include impulsivity; restlessness and hyperactivity; dependency; destructiveness; lack of friends; and immaturity (Chess & Fernandez, 1980; Freeman, 1977; Goldberg, Lobb, & Krou, 1975; Hirshoren & Schnittjer, 1979; Schlesinger & Meadow, 1972). Learning difficulties are also typical in children with hearing loss (Silverman, 1971), and may be a long-term result of the intermittent conductive hearing impairments that result from early chronic otitis media (Brandes & Ehinger, 1981; Downs, 1977; Kaplan, Fleshman, Bender, Baum, & Clark, 1973; Reichman & Healey, 1983).

Linguistic Features

Any hearing loss that involves frequencies of sounds in the range of speech and that occurs during the language acquisition stage seems to result in some abnormality of speech or language development. The extent of this abnormality is, of course, dependent upon both the severity and the duration of the hearing impairment. However, there is no simple one-to-one correlation between severity or duration of hearing impairment and language acquisition. There is some evidence that hearing loss occurring at certain "critical periods" of development (before the age of 3 years) may be associated with later language-learning problems, even if the hearing loss was temporary (Howie, Ploussard, & Sloyer, 1976; Northern & Downs, 1978). Unilateral hearing loss in children may also be associated with language problems. Hearing loss interacts with a number of other factors, such as intelligence and environment, in producing an effect on language acquisition. Hence, there is considerable variability in the types of speech and language acquisition found in children with hearing impairment.

Abnormalities in speech prosody are among the more common speech problems found in children with hearing loss. These prosodic problems include a monotony of pitch and loudness, a tendency for pitch to rise out of control at times, and a harsh voice quality.

Articulatory problems, ranging from isolated defects in the articulation of only a few sounds to speech that is completely unintelligible, have been reported for children with hearing loss. In cases where only a few speech sounds are affected, these are most commonly the high-frequency fricative sounds (/s/, /th/, /sh/, /f/). In cases where articulation defects involve a wide range of sounds, the articulation either may resemble the speech of younger normal children (Oller & Kelly, 1974) or may be completely different from that of normal speakers (Liff, 1973). Articulation problems occur with the production of vowels in the hearing-impaired—something not seen in normals.

In general, there is a strong correlation between amount of hearing loss and amount of expressive language impairment in children (Martin, 1980). Children with hearing loss typically produce shorter sentences and simpler grammar than children with normal hearing (A. Simmons, 1962). The utterances of hearing-impaired children in some ways resemble the "telegraphic" utterances found in young children during language acquisition. A relatively higher proportion of nouns, verbs, and articles, and a relatively lower proportion of adverbs, pronouns, and prepositions, have been demonstrated in the speech of some of these children (Brannon, 1968). The vocabulary of children with hearing loss is often less diverse than that of normal children (Brannon, 1968), although the vocabulary of the hearing-impaired child may be closer to that expected for his age level than his grammar may be (Brenza, Kricos, & Lasky, 1981). There is evidence that the grammatical acquisition of hearing-impaired children differs quantitatively and qualitatively in expression and comprehension from that of normal children (Geers & Moog, 1978; Liff, 1973; West & Weber, 1974).

Although the precise qualitative differences in grammatical acquisition of children with hearing impairment are not understood, it appears that the "higher-level" grammatical structures are among those definitely affected. Even when most of their language acquisition is quite good, children with hearing impairment frequently show difficulties with the comprehension of the subtle refinements in language abilities that are normally acquired after the age of 6 years. One area that seems to present particular difficulty for deaf children is understanding sentences that show a different word order from the typical subject–verb–object order found in English (Quigley, Wilbur, Power, Mantanelli, & Steinkamp, 1976).

Obviously, auditory processing is impaired in children with hearing loss. Some types of hearing loss result in selective impairments in speech perception, such that certain sounds cannot be discriminated, regardless of how loud they may be presented. High-frequency loss in which fricative sounds (such as /s/, /z/, /th/, and /f/) are involved is a good example of this type of hearing loss. Children with high-frequency loss may fail to hear these sounds at all or may perceive (and in turn produce) them all as a /t/ sound.

Children with hearing impairment are interested in communication, and show communicative intent and often highly developed systems of gestures for communication.

Mental Retardation

DSM-III defines "mental retardation" as a condition with onset before age 18 and characterized by general intellectual functioning that is significantly below average (defined by a full-scale IQ score below 70) and by associated impairments in adaptive functioning.

It must be remembered that the diagnosis of mental retardation (like the diagnosis of developmental language disorder) refers not to a single disorder, but rather a class of disorders, the subtypes of which may be very different clinically. DSM-III has defined four subtypes of the disorder: "mild" (or "educable"), "moderate" (or "trainable"), "severe," and "profound." The American Association on Mental Deficiency (1983) manual discusses etiological subtypes.

Nonlinguistic Features

Mental retardation represents a class of disorders that may have resulted from any of a number of different causes, including biological and psychosocial factors. Since in many cases mental retardation is the result of biological factors (e.g., genetic disorders such as Down syndrome, phenylketonuria, or Tay–Sachs disease, or pre- or postnatal traumas such as malnutrition), medical and physical problems are common in mentally retarded children. Among the more common medical problems found in these children are these: physical anomalies; motor and muscular problems (e.g., hypotonia and hyperflexibility of the joints); neurological problems (e.g., seizure disorders, dyspraxia, and early onset of senile brain changes); and visual problems (e.g., myopia, cataracts, and strabismus). Although hearing and responses to sounds are usually normal in mentally retarded children, there is a somewhat greater prevalence of auditory problems in these children than in the general population. It has been estimated that between 15% and 20% of mentally retarded children may have some hearing loss (Fristoe, 1976). Medical disorders of particular relevance with regard to speech and language functioning are hearing loss, oral motor apraxias and dysarthrias, and facial deformities involving the speech mechanism (such as the thickened tongue commonly found in children with Down syndrome).

The motor development and play of mentally retarded children usually resemble those of much younger normal children. Developmental delays in all motor and developmental milestones are typical in mentally retarded children. These children do show appropriate use of objects and toys, although their limited motor coordination and short attention spans may somewhat impair play. These children are often extremely social and outgoing in their play, and particularly enjoy such early games as peek-a-boo.

Associated behavioral problems are common in mentally retarded children, and particularly in younger and lower-IQ children (Ando & Yoshimura, 1978). The most common behavioral problems are hyperactivity and shortened attention span; infantile autism (or symptoms of infantile autism, such as self-injury, withdrawal, stereotyped behaviors, and destructive behaviors); and stereotyped movement disorders.

Linguistic Features

There is, obviously, a relationship between intelligence levels and language acquisition. The greater a child's level of mental retardation, the poorer his language acquisition (Rogers, 1975; Schiefelbusch, 1972). Studies suggest that language impairment is present in 100% of the profoundly retarded, 90% of the severely retarded, and about 45% of the mildly retarded (Carrow-Woolfolk & Lynch, 1982).

This does not mean, however, that all mentally retarded children have similar or uniform reductions in language. The relationship of language development to nonlanguage intelligence level is not a direct one-to-one correlation. It must be remembered, for example, that a disorder in the development of language is not conclusive evidence of low intelligence level, and, conversely, that low intelligence level is not a necessary or sufficient explanation for the inability to talk (Mittler, 1972).

There is considerable clinical evidence that the impairment in language development does not necessarily correspond in degree to the impairment in other abilities found in mentally retarded children. Mittler (1972) states (and our own clinical experience definitely verifies) that it is not at all uncommon to encounter patients with mental ages of 5 years whose language abilities barely reach the 2-year level. There is, in fact, a fairly extensive literature documenting that mentally retarded children in general, and Down syndrome children in particular, seem to be "extra deficient" in verbal tasks

(Luria, 1961; Lyle, 1961; Milgram, 1966; Mittler, 1972). Lillywhite and Bradley (1969), in a survey of mentally retarded children in Portland, Oregon, found that all of the children showed speech and language functioning significantly inferior in one way or another to expectations based upon mental age.

Among mentally retarded children of the same intelligence levels, there can be a wide range of linguistic abilities. Hence, it is difficult to generalize about types of speech and language problems found in mentally retarded children. The communicative problems associated with mental retardation vary in type, severity, and communicative effect (Silverman, 1971). Ryan (1975) states that individual variations in the development of speech and language in mentally retarded children are much greater than those found in normal children.

One statement upon which most authors agree, however, is that articulation problems are among the most prevalent and marked communication disorders found in mentally retarded children (T. Jordan, 1967; Keane, 1972; Spradlin, 1963). Articulation impairments are most prevalent in children with the greatest degrees of retardation (Schiefelbusch, 1972; Spreen, 1965). It has been estimated that articulation defects are present in up to 53% of the mildly retarded and 95% of the more severely retarded (Carrow-Woolfolk & Lynch, 1982). Articulation disorders in mentally retarded children are frequently the result of late neuromuscular development and subsequent poor coordination (Weiss & Lillywhite, 1981). Other common causes of articulation impairments in mentally retarded children include hearing impairment (Fulton & Lloyd, 1968), chronically occluded nasal passages, and deformities of the speech mechanism. Such organic abnormalities may produce abnormal speech prosody, affecting both rhythm and pitch of speech. When there are no organic speech mechanism involvements, articulation errors tend to be of the same type as those found in younger normal children or children with developmental articulation disorder (J. Bangs, 1942; Matthews, 1957).

Abnormalities have also been reported in the speech fluency of mentally retarded children. Stuttering occurs in from 10% to 45% of the retarded; the more severely retarded are less frequently afflicted than the less severely retarded

(Carrow-Woolfolk & Lynch, 1982). Among those not considered stutterers, abnormal speech patterns involving self-repetitions have been reported (Naremore & Dever, 1975).

The language acquisition of mentally retarded children unarguably involves a rate of development slower than that of normal children. Several language studies report that these children exhibit the features of the normal stages of language development found in younger normal children (Graham & Graham, 1971; Ryan, 1975). The language of children with mental retardation usually appears simplified in vocabulary items and sentence structures when compared to the language of normal peers.

There is evidence that mentally retarded children tend to follow a normal pattern of language development, passing through the same stages and sequences of acquisition as do normal children. Lenneberg, Nichols, and Rosenberger (1964), in a language study of mentally retarded children, found a normal pattern of development through the babbling and one-word utterance stages; Lackner (1968) found a normal pattern of development from single words through expanded noun and verb phrases and complex sentences; Yoder and Miller (1972) found a normal order of development of morphological forms; and Semmel and Dolley (1971) and W. Gordan and Panagos (1976) found normal patterns of acquisition for sentence transformations.

Nonetheless, there is also evidence that a type of permanent language deficit, rather than a delay in language development, is involved. For many children with mental retardation, the prognosis for achieving normal language is very poor (Mittler, 1972). Various types of specific deficits in linguistic functioning have been postulated. Several authors have observed specific difficulties with morphological acquisition (Lovell & Bradbury, 1967; Menyuk, 1971; Spradlin & McLean, 1967) or sentence structure (Bliss, Allen, & Walker, 1978; Ryan, 1975; Semmel, Barritt, & Bennett, 1970).

Numerous studies have suggested varied subgroups of mentally retarded children who show different patternings of linguistic performance. D. Chapman and Nation (1981), for example, found six distinct patterns of language performance varying in strength and weakness across such functions as vocabulary, expressive syntax, comprehension of grammar, and syntactic repetition.

Most authors agree that mentally retarded children tend to show deficits in auditory processing. Ensminger and Smith (1965) administered a number of processing tests to mentally retarded children; visual areas (especially visual decoding and visual–motor association) were their greatest strengths, and vocal and auditory encoding were their greatest weaknesses. Rohr and Burr (1978) noted defects in auditory processing, particularly in auditory memory and attention, to be typical of the mentally retarded children they studied.

As suggested above, mentally retarded children use language in a manner typical of younger normal children. These children are friendly, make eye contact, and have the desire to communicate. Gestures (although sometimes limited or simplified) are often used by these children to communicate.

Elective Mutism

Nonlinguistic Features

Children with elective mutism generally have normal medical histories. Kolvin and Fundudis (1981) studied 24 children with elective mutism and found no evidence of consistent neurological, hearing, or perinatal abnormalities. The demographic features of children with elective mutism are also generally unremarkable. The sex ratio in elective mutism is unusual, however: The disorder is at least equally common and perhaps slightly more common in girls than in boys (Kolvin & Fundudis, 1981; Wright, 1968). In Kolvin and Fundudis's (1981) sample, the electively mute children were born significantly early in their sibship. Some authors have reported abnormal family interaction patterns (including parental role reversals, social isolation, overly protective parents, or discordant family relationships) among children with elective mutism (Mayer & Romanini, 1973; Wergeland, 1979), but these findings are not consistent in all studies.

There is some evidence that children with elective mutism have an abnormally high prevalence of other developmental abnormalities. For example, in Kolvin and Fundudis's (1981) study, electively mute children were more apt to have late speech milestones, enuresis, or encopresis than children in the control group. While children with elective mutism as a group are described as having intelligence levels in the normal range, there is some evidence that their average intelligence scores are lower than those of the general population.

The most striking nonlinguistic features of elective mutism have to do with personality and behavior. Children described in the literature have had varying personality features, but most have been characterized as showing some abnormal temperamental features. In Kolvin and Fundudis's (1981) large sample, all of the children showed shyness and failure to communicate verbally in certain circumstances; otherwise, there was a wide variety of personality patterns. Oppositional behavior and poor malleability at home and school were common, ranging from mild to severe. About half of the children in Kolvin and Fundudis's (1981) sample demonstrated a personality pattern of sulky and aggressive behavior; aggression occurred primarily in the home, and sulkiness occurred primarily with strangers. By contrast, 25% of the sample were shy in social situations and relatively submissive at home, and 25% were described as being very sensitive children who cried easily and became easily distressed. In about a third of the cases, children were more withdrawn around peers than around adults, and in 58% of the cases there was an equal withdrawal from peers and adults. In only 8% of cases was the withdrawal greater with adults than with peers.

Kolvin and Fundudis (1981) also found that 29% of the children in their sample had excessive and unusual motor activity. Two of the 24 children were seriously obsessional, one suffered fainting attacks, and one child developed sexual exhibitionism at adolescence. No less than 71% of the group had some associated behavioral problems. It is of note that in the seven cases with motor activity problems, only two had hyperactivity, while five had unusual motor movements (including grimacing and tics).

Linguistic Features

The cardinal feature of elective mutism is abnormal use of spoken language. Electively mute children, although able to talk, speak only with a small group of intimate friends or relatives in very specific situations or environments (usually the home). Although these children rarely speak to strangers or in a clinical setting, it must be noted that they frequently appear friendly, and may communicate long "stories" through (usually) the use of gestures, drawings, or even whispering.

The history of language development is generally normal. Tramer (1934) reports that, prior to the onset of elective mutism, there is no history of speech or language retardation, and various other authors state that elective mutism develops at about the age of 3–5 years after a period of normal speech development (Elson, Pearson, Jones, & Schumaker, 1965; Pustrom & Speers, 1964; Reed, 1963; Salfield, 1950). The mutism may be noticed after the child starts school, and the pattern is that the child speaks at home but not at school.

Language comprehension and expression abilities of children with elective mutism are varied. Most authors agree that a critical diagnostic point is to establish no significant abnormality of language comprehension or production that could explain the mutism. However, it should be noted that Wright's (1968) study revealed that about 20% of the children had an underlying speech or language handicap. In Kolvin and Fundudis's (1981) sample, 50% had immaturities of speech and/or other speech difficulties. Our own research has revealed a number of electively mute children with pervasive underlying language comprehension difficulties.

Organic Articulation Disorders

There are a number of organic conditions involving muscular or neuromuscular disorders or structural abnormalities of the speech mechanism that can produce articulation problems. The majority of these are difficult to remediate and produce more unintelligible speech than does developmental articulation disorder. Nonetheless, milder forms of organic impairment can occur. Space requirements prevent a detailed description of these disorders here, although the three most prevalent conditions found in children are briefly mentioned below. Readers interested in more information about organic articulation disorders are referred to the following works: Aram and Nation (1982), Bloodstein (1979), and Eisenson and Ogilvie (1983).

Cleft Palate

Children with cleft palate show misarticulations of speech sounds, delayed speech milestones, and, in severe cases, delayed language milestones in the early years of life. The speech misarticulations of children with cleft palate tend to be consistent and follow a distinctive pattern: Nasal sounds and semivowels tend to be normal, but stop consonants, fricative consonants, and affricates are abnormal (usually nasal substitutions or distortions). The vocal quality is abnormal; the child with cleft palate has a hypernasal quality and sounds as if he is "talking through his nose." Speech is usually produced with reduced loudness.

Dysarthria

Dysarthria involves some type of disturbance in the control of the speech musculature. Muscular weakness, slow motor movements, limited range of motion, abnormal muscle tone, and abnormal reflexes are usually seen. There may be difficulty starting and stopping motor movements and abnormal posturing. Drooling, slow, or uncoordinated oral motor behavior, and awkward or slow protrusion and retraction of the tongue, may occur. There is usually a history of problems with early feeding, sucking, or chewing in these children, and a family history for similar disorders is often positive. Associated disabilities include language delays, dyslexia, and spelling disability.

The speech of children with dysarthria tends to be slower than normal, with any increase in the rate of speech resulting in a marked breakdown of accuracy. Unlike children with developmental articulation disorder, children with organically based articulation impairments are usually aware of their own misarticulations. Speech misarticulations tend to occur most frequently in consonant clusters, next most frequently in single consonants, and then in diphthongs. Vowels are usually articulated correctly. The speech misarticulations are more frequently distortions or omissions than substitutions, and the errors tend to be consistent. Often it is possible to identify the muscles involved by determining which speech sounds are affected.

Apraxia

Apraxia involves an inability, in the absence of a paresis in the speech musculature, to carry out the voluntary movements required for speech. There are no abnormalities of the motor movements involved in chewing, sucking, or swallowing, but oral movements during speech are awkward and clumsy. Children with apraxia often have a positive family history of apraxia.

Speech misarticulations occur erratically, and consist of reversals of sounds, additions of sounds, and repetitions of sounds, as well as distortions and substitutions. Substitutions may involve phonetically unrelated sounds as well as phonetically similar sounds. Consonants are misarticulated more frequently than vowels, and misarticulations occur more frequently in long sentences or words than in syllables or single monosyllabic words. In younger children, there is usually a markedly restricted repertoire of speech sounds. The disorder can range in intensity from relatively mild to severe. In a severe case, a child may only be able to imitate single sounds in isolation and may not be able to use any sounds for speech. The rate of speech is usually normal, although in severe cases it may be slowed to compensate for the problem. Associated language problems usually are limited to word-finding or expressive skills.

For the differential diagnosis of all organically based articulation disorders, neurological and medical examinations may sometimes be necessary, although in most cases abnormal oral movements or structures will be readily apparent. It must also be remembered that organic articulation impairments can occur in conjunction with developmental articulation impairments (Johnson, 1981).

Childhood Psychoses

Introduction: Conceptualization of the Disorders

"Childhood psychoses" is a global cover term for a heterogeneous group of conditions, including schizophrenia occurring in childhood, childhood schizophrenia, infantile autism, childhood-onset pervasive developmental disorder, and other unspecified syndromes that have been given a variety of names in the literature such as "atypical children." Reviews of the historical aspects of the concept of childhood psychosis can be found in several recent publications (Hassibi & Breuer, 1980; Werry, 1979). In this introduction, we discuss the conceptualization of these disorders and the role that speech and language abnormalities play in their symptomatology.

Childhood Schizophrenia and Schizophrenia Occurring in Childhood

We first consider the schizophrenic disorders. According to DSM-III, the essential features of the schizophrenic disorders include the presence of certain psychotic features such as delusions, hallucinations, incoherence, catatonic behavior, or inappropriate affect during the active phase of the illness; a continuous duration of at least 6 months; and deterioration from a previous level of functioning. The 6-month duration period must include an active phase of at least 2 weeks during which symptoms are present, and may include a prodromal phase (consisting of clear deterioration in function prior to the active phase of the illness), and/or a residual phase (consisting of persistent symptoms following the active phase). Prodromal symptoms, according to DSM-III, may include the following: social withdrawal, impairment in role functioning or personal hygiene, markedly peculiar behavior, bizarre ideation, unusual perceptual experiences, and digressive, vague, incoherent, or circumstantial speech.

DSM-III distinguishes schizophrenia by age of onset: "childhood onset" refers to onset before age 12 years, "adolescent onset" refers to onset between ages 12 and 18, "adult early/mid onset" refers to onset after age 18 and before age 44, and "late onset" refers to onset after age 45 years. Obviously, for developmental reasons, the clinical picture of a child with schizophrenia may be somewhat different from that of an adult with schizophrenia. In the present work, we use two terms to designate the DSM-III diagnosis of schizophrenia when it occurs in children: "schizophrenia occurring in childhood" refers to the disorder occurring in children with essentially the same symptomatology as in adults; and "childhood schizophrenia" refers to the diagnosis when present in children with a different phenomenological picture from that of adults. The frequency of the various symptoms of schizophrenia with regard to age is not well documented, although Beitchman (1983) has reported that thought insertion, thought broadcasting, possession of thought, and emotional blunting, are more frequently found in schizophrenic children than in schizophrenic adults.

The cognitive and linguistic abnormalities that commonly occur in schizophrenic disorders (e.g., delusions, bizarre ideation, incoherence, poverty of speech) have been given the broad term of "thought disorder." Although some early authors (Bleuler, 1950) have regarded thought disorder as pathognomonic of schizophrenia, over the years researchers have questioned the value and specificity of the concept (S. Schwartz, 1982).

The historical antecedents of the term "thought disorder" are well reviewed by Andreasen (1982), who points out that thought processes themselves cannot be observed but only inferred. Hence, she regards the term "thought disorder" as a philosophical term rather than a medical one, and recommends it be avoided in scientific writing. Renaming "thought disorder" as "disorders of thought, language, and communication" (1979, p. 1325), Andreasen enumerates the subtypes as: laconic speech, poverty of content of speech, pressure of speech, distractible speech, tangentiality, derailment, incoherence, illogicality, clanging, neologisms, word approximations, circumstantiality, loss of goal, perseveration, echolalia, blocking, and stilted speech. Andreasen's (1982) work suggests that these categories can be reliably rated, and are not specific to schizophrenia but occur in patients with other psychoses (such as mania) and dementia.

Whether these disorders have the same significance when

they occur in children or adolescents has never been systematically studied, although Beitchman's (1983) review suggests that some of these disorders are relatively common in schizophrenia occurring in childhood. However, there are no normative data on the occurrence of these disorders in children under the age of 5, and no specific data on their occurrence in childhood psychoses. Such data is critical before any diagnostic claims can be made because many of these "disorders" (e.g., perseveration, echolalia, neologisms, word approximations) are common in young normal children.

Clinical Descriptions

LINGUISTIC AND NONLINGUISTIC FEATURES

Unfortunately, no definitive clinical description can be provided for schizophrenia occurring in childhood or childhood schizophrenia, due to the fact that researchers have used these terms (and others dealing with childhood psychoses) in vastly different ways. For example, Howells and Guirguis (1984) have recently reported on 20 patients diagnosed as childhood schizophrenics 20 years earlier. Unfortunately, these patients seem to have been a diverse group diagnostically; their prior diagnoses included infantile autism, pervasive developmental disorder, schizophrenia in childhood, and true childhood schizophrenia. When these children were seen as adults, none were given a diagnosis of schizophrenia using the Schneiderian diagnostic criteria (Schneider, 1959); however all were given a diagnosis of schizophrenia using the Feighner criteria (Feighner *et al.*, 1972).

Another problem for data collection is the rarity of childhood psychoses. Beitchman (1983) has estimated the prevalence of schizophrenia occurring in childhood at less than 0.14 per 1000, almost 50 times less than the prevalence of schizophrenic disorder in adolescents and adults. It appears, however, that the disorder is more prevalent in older children and in males, and possibly in children with a family history of schizophrenia (Hanson & Gottsman, 1976). There is some evidence (Eggers, 1978; Kydd & Werry, 1982) that the younger the age of onset of schizophrenia, the poorer the outcome. However, family history apparently does not exert any impact on outcome (Eggers, 1978; Kydd & Werry, 1982).

Among the characteristics reported in the literature as part of the "preschizophrenic" pattern are problems in relationships, avoidant behavior, withdrawn behavior, school learning problems, behavior problems, magical thinking, and violent temper outbursts.

Pervasive Developmental Disorders

The term "pervasive developmental disorders" as defined in DSM-III refers to disorders that in the past have been called "childhood schizophrenia," "childhood psychosis," "symbiotic childhood psychosis," and other names. These disorders are characterized by distortions in the basic psychological functions involved in the development of social skills and language. The term "childhood psychosis" is not used in DSM-III because these disorders apparently bear little relationship to the traditionally defined psychotic disorders of adult life.

Two specific subtypes of pervasive developmental disorders are described in DSM-III: infantile autism and childhood-onset pervasive developmental disorder. Infantile autism is characterized by core symptoms involving pervasive impairments in reciprocal social interaction, communication, and activities or interests. Childhood-onset pervasive developmental disorder, as originally described in DSM-III, is conceptualized as a residual category. These children do not have schizophrenia occurring in childhood or infantile autism. Their essential features are similar to those of autism, although the diagnostic criteria for autism are not met.

The age-of-onset criteria for these disorders is controversial. Retrospective study of children with childhood-onset pervasive developmental disorder often reveals that insidious symptoms were present before the age of 30 months. Kolvin's (1971) study suggests that onset of any type of psychotic disorder is rare between the ages of 3 and 5 years.

Associated features of childhood-onset pervasive developmental disorder include preoccupation with morbid thoughts; bizarre beliefs; and pathological preoccupation with, and bizarre use of objects. Linguistic features of this disorder, aside from a question-like intonation pattern, lack any detailed description in the literature. In our clinical experience, these children show diverse levels of skills in linguistic areas, their most striking deficits being in the use of language.

Clinical Description of Infantile Autism

NONLINGUISTIC FEATURES

Infantile autism is characterized by major emotional and behavioral features, including a pervasive lack of responsiveness to other people; peculiar interest in or attachments to animate or inanimate objects; resistance to change; aloofness; lack of eye contact; limited physical contact; stereotypic activities, including self-stimulation; shortened attention span and hyperactivity; over- or underattention to stimuli (including failure to show normal responses to pain, abnormal fascination with lights, or apparent deafness); and extreme temper tantrums.

Play, from the earliest records, is deviant. These children fail to show the early imitative games (peek-a-boo, pat-a-cake) that most infants enjoy. Toys generally are used inappropriately. Whether given cars, tools, dolls, blocks, or books, the same primitive patterns of play (putting toys in the mouth, manipulating toys with the hands, arranging toys in patterns, or tossing toys away) will be used. Older autistic children fail to engage in such imaginative play as "school," "house," or "cowboys."

Developmental delays are common in autistic children, and a number of authors have commented on the poor motor coordination skills of autistic children (Bryson, 1970; DeMeyer *et al.*, 1972). Unevenness in development is also common: Cases of autistic children with unexpectedly high development in certain isolated areas have been noted (e.g., Rimland's [1978] reports of "autistic savants" and Huttenlocher and Huttenlocher's [1973] reports on hyperlexic autistic children). Musical abilities in autistic children are often unusually good.

Neurological and medical abnormalities have been cited in a number of autistic children. Rutter (1966) reports that approximately 25% of adolescent autistics develop seizures and approximately 75% of autistic children are mentally retarded. Disorders in voluntary muscle control (particularly oral motor control or apraxic disorders) are present in a number of autistic children (Pronovost, Wakstein, & Wakstein, 1966). Pneumoencephalograms showed left-hemisphere abnormalities in 15 of 17 cases in one study (DeLong, 1978). Gualtieri, Adams, Shen, and Loiselle (1982) report an unusually high frequency of minor physical anomalies in autistic children.

Research studies have revealed cases of paroxysmal EEG abnormalities (Cohen, Caparulo, & Shaywitz, 1976); abnormal cerebral lateralization (Dawson, Warrenburg, & Fuller, 1982); abnormal brain stem auditory evoked potentials (Fein, Skoff, & Mirsky, 1981); neuropathology of the temporal lobes (Hetzler & Griffin, 1981), temporal horn (Hauser, DeLong, & Rosman, 1975), and parietal-occipital region (Hier, Lemay, & Rosenberger, 1979); and biochemical abnormalities involving catecholamine or serotonin levels.

LINGUISTIC FEATURES

Autistic children manifest a wide variety of linguistic deficits. In the most extreme form of the disorder, there may be a complete absence of speech and language. Among those autistic children who are not mute (approximately 50%), disorders involving both speech and language are reported.

The speech of autistic children shows abnormalities in both articulation and prosody; prosodic disturbances are the more severe and lasting (Kanner, 1971; Rutter, 1966). Their speech has been described as "monotonous," "flat," "wooden," "hollow," "sing-song," "hoarse," "harsh," and "hypernasal." In more technical terms, prosodic abnormalities found include limitations in the frequency range of sounds produced and distortions in both speech rhythm and loudness.

The autistic child's speech often contains such articulation errors as the substitution of earlier-acquired for later-acquired sounds and other random or inconsistent substitutions (Shervanian, 1967). Though prevalent in younger autistic children (Savage, 1968; Wing, 1969), articulation errors are frequently transient (Bartak, Rutter, & Cox, 1975) and are less severe than articulation problems found in children with other types of language disorders (Boucher, 1976).

Children with infantile autism invariably present with abnormal histories of language development. The majority have a history of markedly delayed language milestones, although there is a subset of autistic children who present with a history of language development that was reportedly normal and subsequently lost.

Autistic children tend to have limited vocabularies and to use words inappropriately. Kanner (1946) observed a metaphorical or bizarre quality in the language of autistic children. Frequently these children invent their own words, use words with only vague referents or extreme literalness, and develop abnormal vocabularies. Object names are the most easily acquired items for these children, and there are reports of autistic children who develop large vocabularies focusing on a single topic (such as dates, days, times, names of presidents, capital cities, or states) (Kanner, 1946). Abstract words and words with more than one meaning are the most difficult vocabulary items for these children to acquire.

Both the language comprehension and the expressive language of autistic children are defective. Many autistic children are mute; estimates vary from 28% (Lotter, 1967) to 50% (Baltaxe & Simmons, 1975). Estimate variability results from differing definitions of "mutism"; autistic children may be completely silent or may occasionally utter a word or phrase. Although all descriptions of the language of autistic children agree on the presence of grammatical abnormalities, information on the types of grammatical problems is sketchy because of the limited amount of spontaneous speech produced. Most reports note only that autistic children tend to use simplified (often incomprehensible) sentences and few words.

A detailed study of the types of morphemes and sentence structures found in the language of "high-functioning" autistic children, however, revealed that these children's grammatical structures were very similar to those of children with developmental language disorder (Cantwell, Baker, & Rutter, 1978). Among the grammatical problems described by other authors are the following: confusion or reversal of the pronouns "you" and "I" (Kanner, 1946); failure to use other personal pronouns (Hingtgen & Bryson, 1972); failure to use conjunctions (Weiland & Legg, 1964); and difficulty in using verb tense markers correctly (Bartolucci & Albers, 1974).

Some suggest that difficulties in using personal pronouns may be an artifact of sentence position or echolalia (Bartak, Rutter, Cox, & Newman, 1972; Fay, 1971), but it is now believed that this may reflect difficulties in "boundary" references. Autistic children manifest deficits in the use of other concepts, such as "here-there," "come-go," and "bring-take," which involve boundaries and directions. Nouns and imperatives are grammatical structures autistic children seem to have less difficulty using (Weiland & Legg, 1964).

Autistic children demonstrate a discrepancy between verbal-auditory and visual-spatial processing abilities and are superior in the latter. On intelligence tests such as the WISC-R, autistic children invariably perform best on block design or object assembly tasks and poorest on vocabulary or information tasks (J. Simmons & Tymchuk, 1973). Autistics perform poorly on tasks requiring verbal skills even if verbal responses are not required (Rutter, 1978). Abnormal responding to auditory stimuli is often one of the first symptoms reported by parents, who may bring in the children on the suspicion of hearing loss. These children may fail to respond appropriately to sounds as infants, but usually show inconsistent rather than complete absence of response to sounds.

The high levels of functioning and cooperation required by tests of processing abilities, and variability among children, limit the conclusions to be drawn regarding the processing deficits of autistic children. Most authors agree that auditory-visual association or cross-modal processing is severely impaired (Bonvillian *et al.*, 1978; Bryson, 1972; Cowan, Hoddinott, & Wright, 1965; Morton-Evans & Hensley, 1978; Tubbs, 1966). There is also general agreement that autistic children show particular difficulty in dealing with multiple stimuli (Bryson, 1970) and are unable to separate the significant from the redundant features in any (auditory, visual, or motor) modality.

There is confusion regarding the auditory discrimination abilities of autistic children; some authors state that discrimination of speech sounds is intact (Simon, 1975), while others state that auditory discrimination problems, particularly those involving figure-ground distinctions, are common (DeHirsch, 1967). Behavioral observations of autistic children's responses to auditory stimuli tend to support the second position.

Condon (1975) proposes that autistic children may suffer delay in the auditory feedback mechanism, such that they cannot hear themselves correctly. Most authors agree that autistic children show good rote (short-term) memory skills in comparison with their other processing skills, and sometimes in comparison with normal children. These memory skills, however, do not make use of meaning (Frith, 1969; Hermelin, 1971). Hence, when compared to normal children, autistic children tend to show superior skills on memory tasks involving, for example, digit repetition, but show poorer skills for word or sentence repetition. Autistic children's memory also differs in that these children tend to recall better later-presented rather than earlier-presented, items (Boucher, 1981).

Kanner's early (1946) description of autistic children showed abnormal features in language acquisition, language development, and use of language acquired. He reported that language of the autistic child was typified by parroting words and stored phrases without comprehension (immediate or delayed echolalia) and by an absence of original remarks, resulting in inappropriate and noncommunicative interactions.

The echolalia of autistic children has been cited as "the most striking feature of the children's language" (Wolff & Chess, 1965, p. 39). The mere presence of echolalia does not distinguish autistic children; both normal children and children with developmental language disorder go through periods of using a lot of echolalic utterances. However, there is evidence that the type of echolalia used by autistic children differs from that of other children (Cantwell *et al.*, 1978; Pronovost *et al.*, 1966; Shapiro, Roberts, & Fish, 1970). First, delayed echolalia seems to be a more common subtype in autistic children than in normal children. Second, modification of echoed utterances to reflect grammatical acquisition levels is a characteristic of "normal" echolalia rarely seen in autistic echolalia. Furthermore, autistic echolalia is usually characterized by abnormal intonation patterns. Several authors report that the echolalia of autistic children mimics the tones of voice, dialectal characteristics, or even foreign accents of speakers (Carrow-Woolfolk & Lynch, 1982; Ricks & Wing, 1976). It does appear, though, that the echolalia of autistic children represents an attempt at social interactions (Hurtig, Ensnid, & Toblin, 1982; Prizant & Duchan, 1981).

Other aspects of communication that are characteristic of autistic language include lack of questions and informative statements; limited use of gestures; frequent use of imperatives (Hingtgen & Bryson, 1972); lack of normal expressions of curiosity and of responsiveness to changing environmental cues (Wolff & Chess, 1965); frequent use of egocentric utterances, including thinking aloud and inappropriate remarks (Cunningham, 1968); failure to reinforce listeners or to be guided by listener response (Schuler, 1980); endless adherence to a single topic (Ricks & Wing, 1976); and use of "a series of obsessive questions" (Rutter, 1967).

Our research involving detailed linguistic analyses of the spontaneous speech of autistic children (Baker, Cantwell, Rutter, & Bartak, 1976) has revealed that the way in which these children use language structures they have learned is the most striking linguistic feature of infantile autism. Aspects of this unusual usage of language include a decrease in spontaneous remarks; and an increase in delayed echoing, thinking aloud, and action-accompaniment utterances; and inappropriate echoes.

Steps in Establishing a Differential Diagnosis

The cardinal feature of developmental language disorder is limited development in language comprehension or expression. Limited language development may also be present in the Axis I syndromes of elective mutism and schizophrenia occurring in childhood; in the Axis II syndromes of developmental language disorder, developmental articulation disorder, mental retardation, and infantile autism; in a variety of Axis III conditions, including significant hearing loss and various types of organic disorders of the speech mechanism; and, finally, to some degree in the Axis IV condition of psychosocial deprivation. The clinical features associated with each of these syndromes are summarized in Table 4-1.

A step-by-step decision procedure approach to establishing a differential diagnosis in children with abnormal speech or language is presented in Figure 4-1. This figure points to the most likely diagnosis (from among the syndromes that include speech/language abnormalities as part of their symptomatology) to consider in the presence of certain symptomatology or testing results. However, since many of the diagnoses are not mutually exclusive, but in fact tend to co-occur with each other, it is necessary to loop back through the procedure once a diagnosis is obtained to consider the likelihood of other co-occurring diagnoses.

First, in the decision procedure outlined in Figure 4-1, a diagnosis of hearing loss is either established or ruled out on the basis of audiological testing. Second, it is established via interactions, observations of the child interacting with others, or history from the parents, whether the child's use of language for communication is either appropriate or grossly inappropriate. Among these children whose use of language is abnormal, the presence of abnormal eye contact, object usage, social play, and/or gestures, will suggest diagnoses of either pervasive developmental disorder or infantile autism. Among these children whose use of language is normal, the presence of normal eye contact, object usage, social play, and/or gestures, will suggest diagnoses of either elective mutism or schizophrenia. The choice between these two diagnoses may be made on the basis of parental history of language usage that is limited to specific people and places.

For children whose use of language to communicate with others is normal, the next step in the decision procedure is the evaluation of nonverbal intelligence using standardized tests. Those children scoring below 70 on such testing are likely to have the Axis II diagnosis of mental retardation. Conversely, those children scoring above 70 on such testing are more likely to have some type of specific language disorder.

To distinguish among different types of specific childhood language disorders, both a linguistic history and linguistic testing are necessary. Children with a history including sudden onset of linguistic loss most likely have the diagnosis of childhood acquired aphasia. Children who are developmentally abnormal (i.e., do not have a history of sudden linguistic loss) are more likely to have developmental or organic disorders. Such disorders are identified on the basis of the component(s) of language that are affected; impairments in language comprehension indicate a diagnosis of developmental receptive

Table 4-1. Summary of Clinical Features of Different Syndromes Involving Abnormal Language or Speech

Clinical features	Developmental language disorder	Infantile autism	Mental retardation	Developmental articulation	Acquired aphasia
Nonlinguistic features					
Neurological	"Soft signs"	Abnormalities	Some problems	Normal	Abnormal EEG
Hearing	Minor loss	Grossly normal	Some loss	Normal	Normal
Other medical problems	Otitis media	Usually none	Various	None	Hemiplegia
Developmental milestones	Grossly normal	Uneven	Delayed	Grossly normal	Normal
Developmental disorders	Coordination, enuresis	Many	Various	Rarely	None
Nonverbal IQ	Normal or above	Often retarded	Retarded	Normal	Normal
Learning difficulties	Usually present	Present	Present	Sometimes	Present
Clinical psychopathology	Attention deficit, anxiety disorder	Stereotypic, abnormal, aloof, inappropriate	Hyperactivity, stereotyped movements, autistic behavior	Anxiety disorder	Withdrawal
Family history	May be ↑ language disorder	May be slight ↑ autism, ↑ developmental disorder	Depends on cause	May be ↑ speech disorder	Nonspecific
Linguistic Features					
Speech features					
Articulation	Impaired	Impaired	Impaired	Impaired	Impaired
Voice	Normal	Abnormal	Impaired	Normal	Usually normal
Intonation-prosody	Normal	Abnormal	Usually normal	Normal	Usually normal
Fluency	Transient problems	Normal	Usually normal	Transient problems	Usually normal
Language features					
Rate of language development	Slow, abnormal	Slow, abnormal	Very slow	Normal	Stops, then slow
Expressive vocabulary	Limited, anomia	Limited, inappropriate	Limited	Normal	Very limited
Expressive grammar	Limited, deviant	Limited, mute	Limited	Grossly normal	Limited, mute
Receptive vocabulary	Limited or normal	Very limited	Limited	Normal	Limited
Receptive grammar	Limited or normal	Very limited	Limited	Normal	Limited
Auditory processing	Discrimination, memory	Impaired	Impaired	Usually normal	Impaired
Visual processing	Some deficits	Some deficits	Impaired	Normal	Impaired
Echolalia (beyond 3 years	Present	Present, inappropriate	Present	None	Not reported
Inappropriate remarks	Some	Common	Few	None	Not reported
Communicative intent	Present, gestures	Not present	Present	Present	Not reported
Inner language: object use	Normal	Abnormal		Normal	Normal
Inner language: creative play		Absent	Limited	Normal	Not reported
"Thought disorder"	Absent	Absent	Absent	Absent	Absent

Elective mutism	Hearing loss	Organic articu- lation	Schizophrenia occurring in childhood	Pervasive developmental disorder
Normal	Normal	Abnormalities	Generally normal	Generally normal; "soft signs"
Normal	Abnormal	Abnormal	Normal	Normal
None	Various	Oral motor	Nonspecific	Nonspecific
Grossly normal	Slight delays	Delays	Grossly normal	Varies
Enuresis, encopresis	Learning only	Various	May have learning disorders	Varies
Normal	Normal	Grossly normal	Generally normal; subgroup with low IQ	Generally normal
Sometimes	Present	Present	Often present	May be present
Shyness	Various problems, withdrawal	Some problems	Often avoidant and shy, hallucinations, ideas of reference	Gross relationship abnormality plus other specific symptoms
↑ Psychopathology (nonspecific)	Depends on cause	Nonspecific	↑ Schizophrenia in parents	Nonspecific
Mute-normal	Impaired	Impaired	Generally normal	Generally normal
Mute-normal	Abnormal loud- ness	Abnormal	Generally normal	Generally normal
Mute-normal	Abnormal pitch	Abnormal	Generally normal	Question-like melody
Mute-normal	Normal	Grossly normal	Generally normal	Generally normal
Normal, slow	Slow	Slow-normal	Generally normal	Slow-normal
Mute-normal	Limited	Limited-normal	Normal	Use of language abnormal
Mute-normal	Limited	Limited-normal	Normal	Use of language abnormal
Mute-normal	Limited	Limited-normal	Normal	Varies
Mute-normal	Limited	Limited-normal	Normal	Varies
Mute-normal	Impaired	Impaired	May be impaired	May be impaired
Mute-normal	Impaired	Grossly normal	Grossly normal	Grossly normal
None	None	None	None	Possible
None	Few	None	May be present	Varies
Present, nonverbal	Normal	Normal	Not reported	Abnormal
Normal	Normal or slightly delayed	Normal	Normal	Normal
Normal	Normal or slightly limited	Normal	Normal	Normal
Absent	Absent	Absent	Present	Absent

Figure 4-1. Decision procedure for differential diagnosis of childhood speech/language disorder.

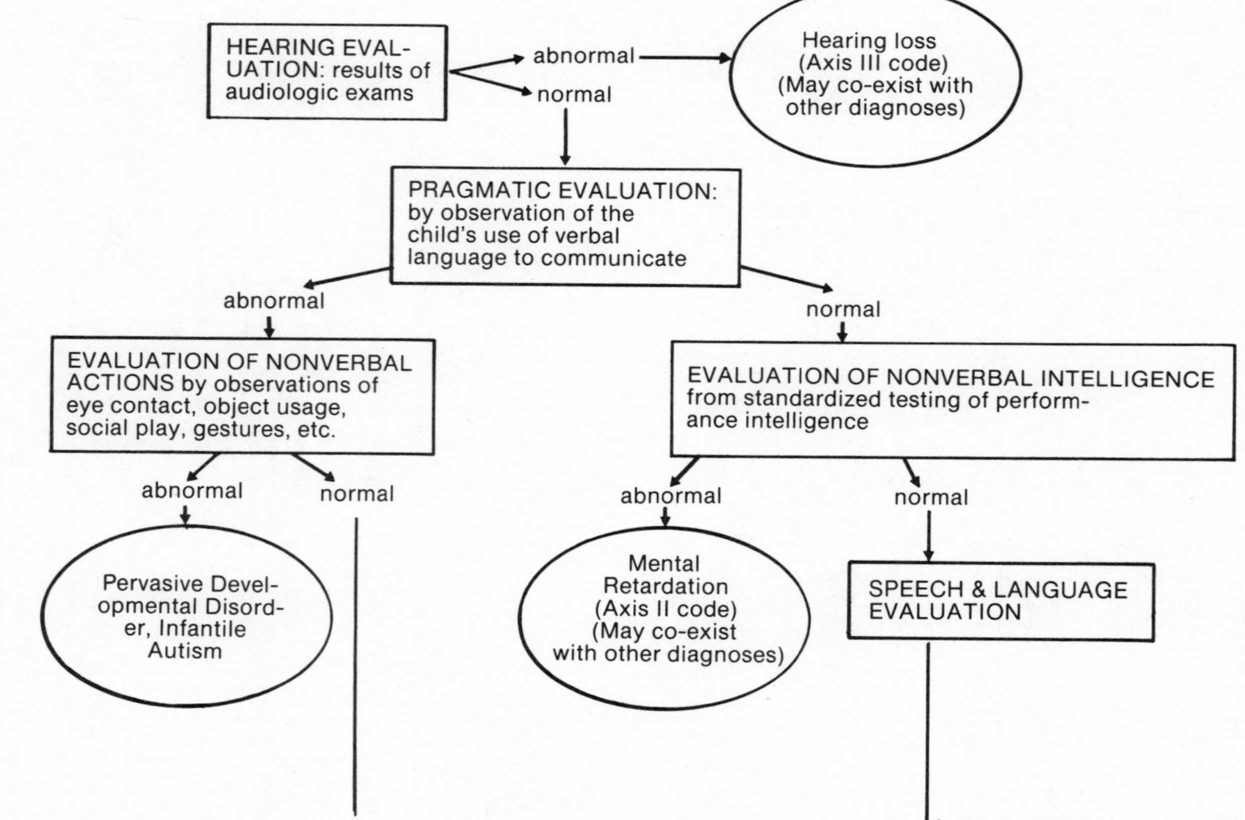

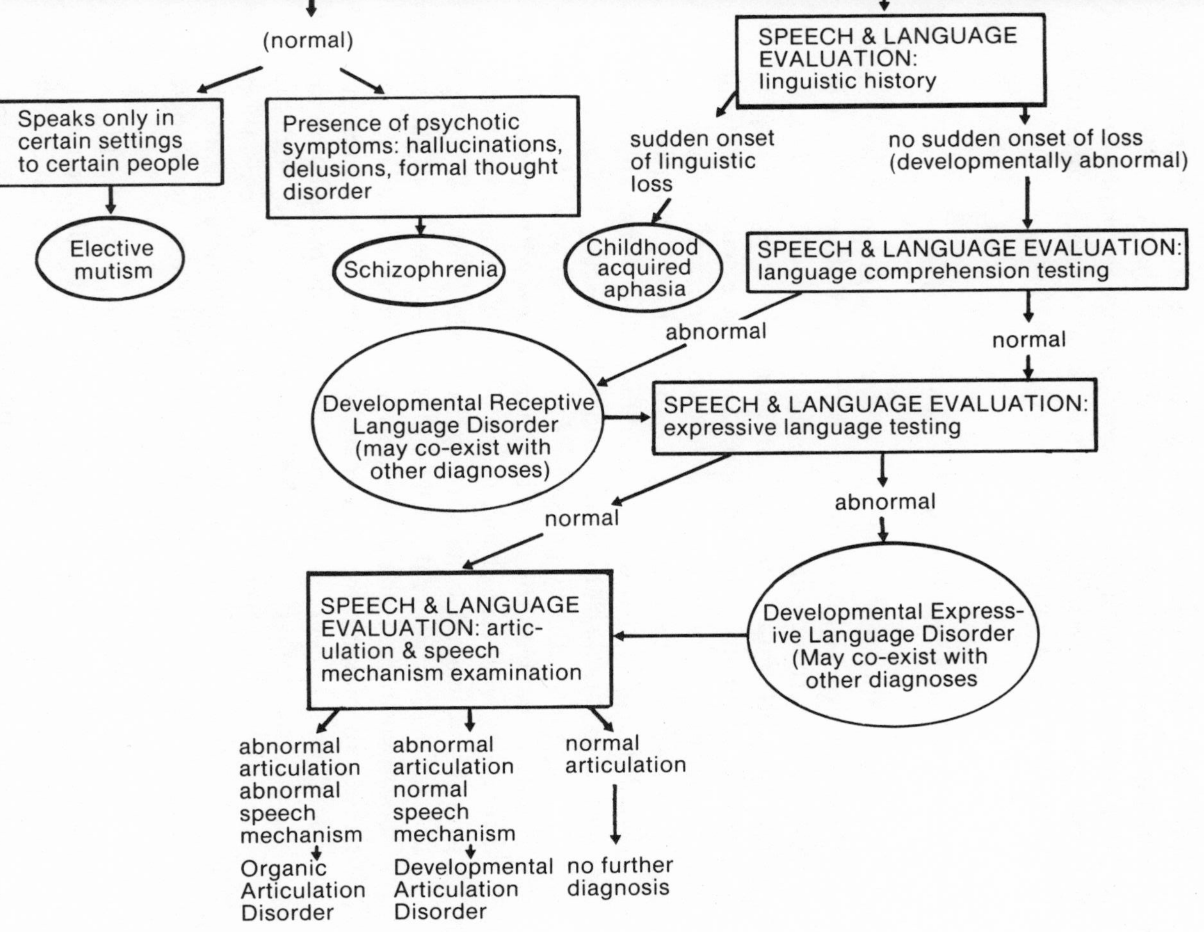
(normal)
Speaks only in certain settings to certain people
Elective mutism
Presence of psychotic symptoms: hallucinations, delusions, formal thought disorder
Schizophrenia
SPEECH & LANGUAGE EVALUATION: linguistic history
sudden onset of linguistic loss
Childhood acquired aphasia
no sudden onset of loss (developmentally abnormal)
SPEECH & LANGUAGE EVALUATION: language comprehension testing
abnormal
normal
Developmental Receptive Language Disorder (may co-exist with other diagnoses)
SPEECH & LANGUAGE EVALUATION: expressive language testing
normal
abnormal
Developmental Expressive Language Disorder (May co-exist with other diagnoses)
SPEECH & LANGUAGE EVALUATION: articulation & speech mechanism examination
abnormal articulation abnormal speech mechanism
Organic Articulation Disorder
abnormal articulation normal speech mechanism
Developmental Articulation Disorder
normal articulation
no further diagnosis

language disorder; impairments in expressive language indicate a diagnosis of developmental expressive language disorder; impairments in speech articulation indicate a diagnosis of either developmental or organic articulation disorder. A change between DSM-III and DSM-IIIR is that, in DSM-IIIR, the various types of developmental speech and language disorders are specifically conceptualized as being nonmutually exclusive, and generally co-occurring, diagnoses.

Tools in Establishing a Multiaxial Diagnosis

The steps outlined in Figure 4-1 for distinguishing between those syndromes involving speech/language abnormalities use information from a variety of different sources including formal speech/language testing, audiological testing, intelligence testing, and history. In addition, (as will be discussed in Chapter 6), children with speech/language abnormalities are very likely to have other DSM-III Axis I psychiatric disorders and Axis II learning disorders, and additional information may be needed to establish these additional diagnoses.

In general, the diagnosis of Axis I clinical psychiatric syndromes is made on the basis of the interview with the parents, interviews with and observations of the child, and the use of parent and teacher behavioral rating scales. Since Axis I syndromes are, in general, clinical diagnoses, it is rare that any laboratory studies, physical exams, or neurological exams contribute to making the diagnosis. For Axis II developmental disorders, however, the diagnosis is generally made by history and by psychometric or other specialized testing, including speech/language tests, intelligence tests, and educational achievement tests. Axis III physical conditions are generally diagnosed on the basis of history, physical exam, neurological exam, and appropriate laboratory studies.

In establishing the multiaxial diagnosis, a variety of tools can be used. There are standardized interviews of a semistructured nature that can be done with parents and with children that aid in the making of Axis I and Axis II diagnoses. Among the most prominent are the Diagnostic Interview for Children and Adolescents (DICA) (Welner, 1985) and the Diagnostic Interview Schedule for Children (DISC) (Radloff, 1985). Both of these are interviews that have a child version and a parent version, are semistructured, and are designed to elicit the symptomatology of the common childhood and adolescent psychiatric syndromes. Another semistructured interview, with both parent and child versions is the Kiddie-SADS (Puig-Antich, 1985), which focuses on more intensive evaluations of children with affective symptomatology and is somewhat less helpful with other psychiatric disorders.

Useful behavioral rating scales include the parent and teacher scales of Achenbach (1978) and Conners and Barkley (1985), and the child self-rating scales of Achenbach (1985) and Beitchman (1985). Originally developed for use in drug studies, the Conners parent and teacher scales focus on hyperactivity, attention deficit, and overt behavior disorders. The Child Behavior Profile for parents and teachers (Achenbach, 1978), on the other hand, covers a broader range of psychopathology, and have more detailed normative data. Both of the child self-rating scales cited are broad range scales designed to elicit many aspects of psychopathology; Beitchman's designed for younger children, and Achenbach's designed for older children and adolescents.

A comprehensive discussion and review of these and other psychiatric evaluation instruments including interviews with children, interviews with parents, observation scales, and parent and teacher rating scales may be found in Rutter, Tuma, & Lann (in press). Other tools that may be employed in psychiatric evaluation include projective psychological tests, physical exams, and neurological exams. While projective psychological tests may have some value as clinical instruments to elicit certain types of material from children, their value from the psychometric standpoint in making specific DSM-III diagnoses in children is somewhat less than well established. Physical exams (including laboratory work such as X-rays and blood studies) and neurological exams are generally not useful in making DSM-III Axis I diagnoses. However, they are helpful in some cases. For example, a child with an organic syndrome secondary to petit mal epilepsy may present with a confusing picture that includes symptoms suggestive of an attention deficit disorder. In such a case, physical and neurological exams including EEG will help clarify the correct diagnosis.

CHAPTER 5

Case Illustrations

Introduction

This chapter contains three case illustrations of children who had various difficulties involving speech and language development. Each case presentation is set up so that the reader can proceed through a typical evaluation—beginning with presenting complaints and history, then the selection of methods of evaluation, then the obtaining of test results, and finally the establishment of a differential diagnosis. The significance of each case is also discussed. The cases selected include a typical child with developmental language disorder (B., discussed second); a more unusual case of a child with a developmental language disorder involving only narrow aspects of language development (J., discussed first); and a child with pervasive developmental disorder (S., discussed last).

Case Illustration: "J."

Presenting Complaints and History

J. was a 14-year-old boy who presented for speech and language evaluation with a history of learning problems, early speech and language delay, rather bizarre and inappropriate use of language, and significant behavior problems at home.

J.'s mother reported that his behavior in school and behavior at home were quite different. At school, J. was a model student in terms of behavior (although he had significant learning problems), whereas at home, J.'s behavior was described as "simply impossible."

The process of the evaluation consisted of a detailed history from both parents; interviews and observations of J.; the use of parent and teacher behavior rating scales; physical and neurological examinations; and speech, language, and achievement testing. J.'s parents brought his baby book, numerous school report cards, and previous medical and psychological evaluations, and thus were able to provide a very detailed history.

In the area of speech and language, J.'s early developmental history showed delays. He said his first word, "hi," at the age of 18 months, and his other language milestones were also late. He was always much harder to understand than other children his age. At the age of 4, speech therapy was initiated three times a week and continued until J. entered school. Thus, J. apparently suffered from articulation and expressive language problems when younger; however, the history did not suggest current problems in these areas. A psychiatrist who had seen J. 1 year prior to our evaluation thought that J. might have "prepsychotic tendencies." This diagnosis was apparently based upon J.'s bizarre remarks and inappropriate use of language.

Aside from the delayed speech and language development, J.'s early history was unremarkable. He was the product of a normal pregnancy, but his delivery was complicated by the use of forceps, resulting in a fractured clavicle. As a neonate, J. was quiet and passive but happy, and he was contented observing his toys. He ate and slept well and was characterized by his mother as a "perfect baby." There was nothing in his past or present history to suggest abnormal responses to sounds, visual deficits, or motor deficits. His motor milestones were normal. J.'s mother had kept detailed notes on his development as part of a project in a child development class. He regarded faces at 3 weeks, made a fist at 4 weeks, followed eyes at 5 weeks, recognized a bottle at 12 weeks, regarded his mobile and clutched at a toy at 15 weeks, cooed at 14 weeks, laughed at 20 weeks, sat and leaned at 25 weeks, vocalized at toys at 30 weeks, sat alone at 38 weeks, held a bottle at 40 weeks, and walked with help at 52 weeks.

There was an early history of "hyperactive behavior" at

17 months, when J. first began to walk alone. From that point on, according to J.'s mother, he would never sit still—not for television, not for books, and not to play games. The pediatrician noted that at age 3, J. did look "hyperactive," but no official diagnosis was made. At the age of 4 years, intellectual testing revealed normal intelligence overall, but skills ranged from the 1½-year-old level to the 4½-year-old level. The lowest scores were in verbal communication and fine motor coordination.

Learning problems appeared in first grade, when J. was identified as not being "reading ready." At this time he was placed in a special learning disability class. Four intelligence tests were administered by different school psychologists over time, but all revealed full-scale IQs in the range of 80–90. Hearing and vision were always found to be normal when evaluated. Genetic work-up revealed no history of heritable biological abnormalities. Several neurologists had seen J. at different points in time. One found an abnormal EEG with some excessive spindling, but there was no clinical evidence of underlying seizure disorder or of any disease or damage to the nervous system.

At the age of 6, when J. was placed in the special class for learning-disabled children, he was also prescribed stimulant medication for hyperactivity. Both the special classes and the medication had continued throughout J.'s school career, and at the time of our evaluation, J. was taking 20–45 milligrams of methylphenidate daily. J.'s mother felt the medication was "not particularly helpful," possibly because of the dosage schedule (morning and noon dosage).

J.'s current teacher rating scale and report card indicated moderate to severe learning problems, but no behavioral complaints. J. was functioning in arithmetic and spelling at about the fourth-grade level, in English at about the fifth-grade level, and in reading at about the sixth-grade level. The teacher stated, "In his self-contained learning-disabled class, J. functions well. He is helpful, considerate of others, willing to attempt any task assigned to him, and able to maintain attention throughout his classes. He is liked by the students in our class and has even been elected class president. He has good relationships with teachers and is liked by all adults who have come in contact with him in the school. Outside of the class, however, he tends to stay by himself.

J.'s behavioral picture at home was quite different. On the parent rating scale and in the parent interview, both the mother and the father detailed a number of complaints. These included overt behavioral symptoms such as impulsivity, inability to concentrate or pay attention for long periods of time, excessive demands for attention, getting in many fights, using obscene language, having a hot temper, talking back, blaming others for his mistakes, having a "short fuse," and showing a low frustration tolerance. In addition to overt behavioral symptomatology, the parents reported emotional symptomatology, including abnormal fears and feelings of inferiority. Neither the mother nor the father gave any history suggestive of hallucinations, delusions, or obsessive–compulsive behavior. There was no clear history of sustained depressive mood disturbance, but the parents mentioned times when J. seemed to be "more hyper than he usually is." These times, however, could not be clearly defined as manic episodes.

Overall Approach to the Evaluation

It was clear from the history of late first-word milestone and early difficulties in being understood that J. suffered from both articulation and expressive language problems when he was younger. The current history did not suggest problems in either of these areas. However, the family history and achievement tests were suggestive of some type of underlying disorder in language comprehension or language processing.

The family history was contributory, in that J. was a late third-born child in a family with multiple other problems. The father was a high school teacher, and there was a 26-year-old brother and a 20-year-old sister. Both brother and sister were currently employed as clerks in a small store, having graduated from high school despite significant problems with learning in childhood. J.'s sister had been hospitalized in her midteens for what might have been a psychotic episode. There were three paternal nephews, all with significant learning disabilities and hyperactivity, and two paternal uncles with learning disabilities and "emotional problems," the nature of which was unclear. Thus, hyperactivity, problems with attention and concentration, and learning difficulties were present not only in J., but also in a number of his close relatives. These problems are frequently associated with disorders of language comprehension and/or auditory processing.

There was a reported discrepancy between the verbal and nonverbal portions of J.'s intelligence testing. This also was suggestive of comprehension or language-processing problems. The main focus of J.'s evaluation thus was on language, learning, and his behavioral and emotional difficulties.

Procedures Selected and Data Collected

SPEECH PRODUCTION, EXPRESSIVE LANGUAGE, RECEPTIVE LANGUAGE, AND USE OF LANGUAGE

In order to try to obtain some clues as to the justification for J.'s earlier diagnosis as "prepsychotic," as well as to put J. at ease, the evaluation began informally with general conversation and "mental status examination"-type questions. This permitted informal assessment of responses to sounds, speech production, expressive language, use of language, and pragmatics.

During the informal interview as well as during the structured psychiatric interview, J. denied any problems. Throughout the interview, he showed very poor attention span and markedly impulsive and irritable behavior. There were no hallucinations evident, and J. appeared alert and well oriented to time, place, and person.

J.'s speech was rapid and fluent. He tended to have somewhat immature speech patterns, and made frequent circumstantial remarks. There were no clear-cut deficits in either vocabulary or comprehension of spoken language. J. gave some inappropriate or tangential responses to certain questions, which caused the examiner to wonder about his comprehension, but there was no clear pattern evident in these inappropriate responses.

AUDITORY PROCESSING AND SEMANTIC DEVELOPMENT

In order to assess J.'s auditory memory, auditory reasoning, and semantic acquisition, the "auditory attention span," "verbal absurdities," "verbal opposites," and "likenesses and differences" subtests of the DTLA[1] were administered. J. scored well below age level on all of these subtests. However, the most interesting findings were not J.'s subtest scores, but the types of responses he gave during the various subtests. Almost all of the subtests showed irrelevant and puzzling responses. Some examples are provided below:

EXAMINER: I'm going to read you something that's silly, and I want you to tell me what's wrong with it. O.K.?: "A little child was drowning in the middle of the lake. His mother shouted to her friends, 'Don't stand there doing nothing. Bring me my rubbers so that I may rescue my child.'" What's wrong with that?

J.: She can't rescue her child because she is drowning.

EXAMINER: Who is drowning?

J.: The mother.

EXAMINER: Here's another one: "Early in the morning, as soon as he finishes supper, my father reads the morning paper." What's wrong with that?

J.: You read the dinner paper, not the morning paper.

EXAMINER: What's the opposite of "same"?

J.: "Insane."

EXAMINER: What's the opposite of "lend"?

J.: "Take off."

EXAMINER: What's the opposite of "former"?

J.: "Casual."

EXAMINER: I'm going to say some words and I want you to say them back to me: "Stone, blot, freeze, vase, ink, toad."

J.: "Stone, blot, froze, raise, pink, coke."

1. For this and other abbreviations of tests and scales used in these cases, see Chapter 3, Appendix C.

EXAMINER: What should you do if you're playing near a place where someone is very sick?

J.: Land.

EXAMINER: What?

J.: You should land your plane so it wouldn't disturb them.

EXAMINER: What should you do if you get a letter with "RSVP" on it?

J.: Return it to the police.

EXAMINER: Do you know what "RSVP" means? It's French for "Respond, please."

J.: Oh, I didn't know that. Then you should answer the letter.

EXAMINER: What's the difference between a physician and a surgeon?

J.: A physician is a place and a surgeon is a doctor who operates.

EXAMINER: What's the difference between a canal and a river?

J.: They both have to do with water, but a canal is made out of wood.

EXAMINER: What's a canal?

J.: I don't know, it's some kind of boat Indians make.

EXAMINER: What's the difference between ignorance and stupidity?

J.: They're both rather fast, but ignorance is anxious and stupidity is something dumb.

EXAMINER: What does it mean to "put the cart before the horse"?

J.: That's slowing down the horse.

EXAMINER: What does it mean to "see eye to eye"?

J.: We look at each other straight in the eyes.

EXAMINER: What does it mean to "talk shop"?

J.: To talk real loud, like "hi" (*said in a deep voice*).

EXAMINER: What does it mean to "burn the candle at both ends"?

J.: That's very bad. You're supposed to burn the wick end and hold the other end; if you burned the end you hold, you'd get hurt.

LEARNING

J. tested at third-grade level in achievement on both the Wide Range Achievement Test (Jastak, Bijou, & Jastak, 1976) and the Gray Oral Reading Tests (Gray, 1967). During the reading test, J. frequently misread words. This resulted in J.'s reading often being a senseless garble, although he did not seem aware of it. J.'s responses to reading comprehension questions were frequently guesses based upon general information about the world, rather than responses specific to the text he had just read. J.'s spelling was also garbled and only vaguely resembled the correct words.

Some examples of J.'s reading and spelling test performance are provided below:

Sentences to read	*J.'s reading*
He is his own mechanic.	He is on machines.
Anyone who encounters difficulty . . .	Anyone who can enter difficulty . . .
He faces real dangers.	He forces real dangers.
Inside were long counters.	Inside were long countries.

Stimulus word	*J.'s spelling*
correct	crearret
material	meartrial
literature	litture
purchase	purshess
decision	dission
opportunity	oppturned

INTERVIEW BEHAVIOR

J. presented an interesting picture in interview: There were times when his conversational language did seem to be "off the wall." He admitted to a large number of separation fears and some generalized anxiety symptomatology. He denied any hallucinations or delusions, and also denied any sustained periods of depression, mania, or manic-like behavior; however, he did admit to interpersonal problems in the home, primarily involving oppositions to his mother and father. As he stated,

"Sometimes I don't keep the rules." He denied significant problems with attention, impulsivity, and motor activity in the classroom setting, and claimed that the medication he was taking "doesn't do anything for me."

Discussion and Differential Diagnosis

J.'s test results showed that, typical of many older language-disordered children, he had problems with sentence structure, with abstract and/or idiomatic word usage, and with the usage of words in unfamiliar contexts. The terms "ignorance" and "stupidity" were only vaguely grasped by J., as were all of the idiomatic expressions given, and he was completely thrown by the use of the expression "morning paper" because he was only familiar with an evening paper.

J.'s lack of skills in auditory discrimination and in sentence structure were reflected in his spelling performance and his reading, where he appeared unable to recognize garble from the "real thing." J.'s linguistic performance at the rather advanced age of 14 showed such marked impairment in auditory discrimination and understanding of abstract concepts that it was alarming to speculate on what his level of functioning at a younger age would have been. Apparently a large portion of what J. heard about the world must have indeed been garbled to him. It was little wonder, then, that he was unable to distinguish garble in his oral reading.

J. was also hampered by his severe attentional problems when he was not on his psychostimulant medication. The teacher's report indicated that he was better in this regard when treated with the proper dose of psychostimulants. However, J. took his medication on an erratic basis, because he himself did not think it did anything for him.

J. had been seen in the past by a number of treating physicians, some of whom used phenothiazines, which did not have the positive effect on his attention span in the classroom setting that the stimulants did. It is most likely that J. was treated with phenothiazines because his language at times made him appear "psychotic." However, it appeared, based on this evaluation, that the language abnormalities reflected underlying auditory discrimination problems and not psychosis.

Although many of J.'s responses did appear to be totally "off the wall," it was clear upon careful analysis that they were the result of incorrect perceptions on his part. Apparently, J. thought that the words he was being asked the opposite of were "sane" rather than "same," "land" rather than "lend," and "formal" rather than "former." J. also misperceived "playing" as "plane," "RSVP" as "police," "physician" as "position," and "canal" as "canoe."

In summary, on Axis I of DSM-III, J. showed a lifelong history of attention deficit disorder with hyperactivity, which was being successfully treated (at least from the classroom standpoint) with the proper dose of psychostimulant medication. However, J. took this only erratically, and the dosage schedule (morning and noon) meant that the medication was not present in the after-school period, when the parents observed him. Also on Axis I, J. presented with some separation fears and symptoms of generalized anxiety, but they were not causing any significant functional impairment, particularly in comparison to his other problems.

On Axis II, J. showed a deficit in areas of language development and processing, doubtless the residual effects of his earlier developmental language disorder. The early developmental articulation problem was no longer present, but there were mixed specific learning problems. There were no history or test data to suggest infantile autism, pervasive developmental disorder, or mental retardation.

On Axis III, there was no evidence of current physical or neurological disorders that were contributing to his developmental language disorder or to his attention deficit disorder with hyperactivity.

On Axis IV, there was a strong family history of attention and learning disorders in close family members, and there was some evidence of disturbed family interaction, secondary to J.'s oppositional behavior and the parents' response to that.

From the treatment standpoint, J. appeared to require a comprehensive treatment program aimed at his learning difficulties, his language problems, and his attention deficit disorder. All of these disorders were interacting to produce a complex picture that was causing J. a great deal of functional impairment, both in the academic setting with regard to learning and in the home setting with regard to his behavior.

Case Illustration: "B."

Presenting Complaints and History

B. presented for evaluation at age 3 years, 8 months, as a result of referral from his nursery school teacher. The teacher had first recommended evaluation when B. was 3 years old for suspected "neurological problems, possibly seizures." At that time, B. had received a neurological evaluation and had been found to have no abnormalities. Subsequently, the teacher had still insisted that something was wrong and had insisted on further evaluation.

The mother reported that, although B. was "behind in language, and a little slow in everything," he was, in both her opinion and the opinion of her pediatrician, "a normal child." Upon probing, however, "some minor problems" were mentioned—chiefly, inability to separate from the mother at the beginning of each school day (manifested by clinging to the mother, crying, and ignoring the other children for the first hour or so); additional clinging when the mother picked him up after school; and tantrums whenever the parents tried to leave B. with a babysitter.

The teacher had written a long letter discussing her concerns about B. She stated that although she had been teaching B. for 7 months, and had seen considerable improvement in his functioning during that time, she was still extremely concerned about his behaviors. She described the daily difficulty in separating from the mother, which she assessed as being "more out of fear than a true temper tantrum." Also, at the beginning of school, B. rarely participated in activities; he might typically be found moving cars from one side of the room to the other and lining them up in an almost perseverating fashion.

The teacher reported that B. rarely spoke, and when he

did, his speech was "imitative of intonation without being imitative of words." There was some question as to how much B. was aware of the school procedures; for example, when it was time to go home or to leave one activity for another, B. would just sit there looking as though he had no idea what was expected of him. Nonetheless, the teacher observed that at times B. communicated nonverbally with the other children, and they seemed to like him.

The medical and developmental history was unremarkable. B. was the product of a normal, full-term pregnancy and birth. There were no feeding problems, and developmental milestones were as follows: sitting at 6 months; crawling at 8 months; standing at 8 months; walking aid at 11 months; walking alone at 15 months; self-feeding at 11 months; self-dressing at 36 months. B. had pneumonia at 2 years 6 months of age, but no other medical problems.

The mother did not recall any abnormalities regarding speech or hearing during infancy, but reported that B. "simply didn't talk at all" until the age of 18 months. From age 18 months, when B. said his first word, to his second birthday, B. only acquired three words, although he seemed to understand "about 10 words." From his second birthday on, only a few more words were acquired, and their articulation was poor and did not improve over time. When B. was 2½ years of age, the mother had taken him to the pediatrician to discuss the poor speech, but the pediatrician had labeled the mother "an overconcerned parent" and had assured her that the child was normal. Prior to his third birthday, no one except the family members could understand B.'s speech. The mother stated that she believed that teasing and ridicule by other children had caused B.'s limited use of language and failure to acquire new words.

Overall Approach to the Evaluation

It was clear from B.'s history that he suffered from deficits in speech and language. Both the past history and the current complaints suggested speech and language performance that was significantly below the level expected for the chronological age levels. The pediatrician's assessment of B. at age 2½ years as a "normal child," when he could not be understood outside the family setting, was highly suspect.

The teacher's description of the solitary, fearful child—unable to separate from his mother, rarely speaking, unaware of basic school routines, and sometimes "just sitting there" or playing in perseverative fashion—could indeed indicate a seizure disorder. However, in view of the normal neurological examination, other diagnoses such as mental retardation, hearing impairment, receptive language disorder, anxiety disorder, pervasive developmental disorder, and even elective mutism had to be considered.

Procedures Selected and Data Collected

COMPREHENSION, COGNITION, AND BEHAVIOR

B. separated from his mother with some difficulty, and was slow to warm up to the examiners. After the initial upset about leaving the mother, B. relaxed and gradually appeared contented drawing or playing with blocks, looking at books, or otherwise engaging in solitary play. His attention span for such tasks was normal or better, and his motor skills (in drawing lines, circles, and simple pictures, and in building block towers) were superior for his age. He was also able to correctly perform oral motor actions such as blowing, sticking out his tongue, and moving his tongue from side to side. Responses to sounds were normal. Use of toys was appropriate, but no spontaneous interactions with the toys occurred.

After a long period of play and warm-up, the examiners were able to get B. to engage in following instructions and doing some formal testing. His cooperation at following commands or answering questions was highly intermittent, and hence it was difficult to estimate his levels of functioning. He performed correctly about half of the simple commands he was given (e.g., "Give me the book," "Put the book on the table," "Pick up the book," "Open the book"), but he ignored the other commands given.

B.'s cooperation was limited for testing, with excessive

amounts of encouragement being needed in order to elicit any responses. It was not possible to obtain intelligence testing scores, but the PPVT was administered, and a score of 2 years, 1 months was obtained. These results were reviewed with the mother, who confirmed that the items that B. had missed on the test ("cone," "baking," "river," "ringing," "ladder," "tire," "snake," "nail," and "jacket") were all words that he did not know. During the administration of this test, B. would at times stop responding in midtask and stare as if not comprehending the task, even though he had previously performed satisfactorily.

SPEECH PRODUCTION, EXPRESSIVE LANGUAGE, AND LANGUAGE USE

B.'s spontaneous speech was limited. Within the first half hour of evaluation, only occasional isolated words were used ("no," "Mommy," and "gimme"). When he wanted some object, B. would point to it. However, when that behavior failed to obtain the desired object for him, he would attempt to name it while pointing and gesturing. Unfortunately, many of his names were not intelligible without the accompanying gestures. For example, "gun" was "duh," "scissors" was "duhduh," and "fish" was "pet."

Even after he warmed up, B.'s responses were very limited. He did state his name, but he held up his fingers to show his age, and generally only pointed to objects when he was asked what they were. Adding to the difficulty in interpreting B.'s remarks was the fact that B. occasionally misnamed items. For example, he called a squirrel "wa" ("rabbit"), and a shovel "di" ("dig"). The majority of B.'s utterances were single words, although there were occasional two-word combinations—for example, "dye do" (which meant "tie my shoe"), and "me dough" (which meant "I am going now").

Discussion and Differential Diagnosis

B.'s history of delays in reaching early speech and language milestones, and of behavioral problems in school, were typical of a child with receptive language difficulties. The inability to follow simple commands, to name objects correctly, to formulate longer sentences, and to articulate sounds accurately are all typical linguistic features of developmental language disorder.

B.'s normal or advanced developmental milestones, motor skills, and play skills all ruled out mental retardation as an explanation for his speech difficulties. Although his articulation was very defective, it could be seen that there was also difficulty in using the proper words and in constructing sentences. This ruled out developmental articulation disorder as the sole explanation for the problem, and suggested a developmental language disorder. B.'s inability to follow commands indicated that there was receptive as well as expressive impairment. Thus, B.'s Axis II diagnosis would be developmental language disorder involving expressive language, receptive language, and speech articulation.

In addition to his developmental language disorder, B. presented with a number of behavioral and emotional abnormalities that required differential diagnosis. These included anxiety symptoms, temper tantrums, some perseverative and solitary behavior, and lack of participation in school activities, all of which might indicate a pervasive developmental disorder such as infantile autism.

The evaluation of these problems with parent interviews, observations of B., and parent and teacher rating scales showed that the anxiety symptoms were predominantly related to separation from those individuals (such as the mother) to whom B. was attached. There was no history of more generalized and persistent anxiety, of persistent shrinking from familiarity or contact with strangers, or of irrational avoidance of objects or situations. Thus the diagnoses of overanxious disorder, avoidant disorder, simple phobia, and social phobia were ruled out. B.'s Axis I diagnosis was separation anxiety disorder. Since B.'s temper tantrums only occurred in conjunction with separation experiences, no behavior disorder diagnoses (such as oppositional, conduct, or attention deficit disorders) were made.

Although B. demonstrated some isolative and perseverative behavior, he did not have true obsessions or compulsions. He did demonstrate the capacity for warm, satisfying interpersonal relationships in the home, and thus schizoid disorder was ruled out. Moreover, infantile autism or another pervasive developmental disorder was clearly not present, as B. did not present with a pervasive lack of responsiveness to others that had been present for a sustained length of time, nor did he have multiple bizarre behaviors.

Thus the final diagnoses were developmental language disorder and separation anxiety disorder.

Follow-Up Evaluation

INTERVAL HISTORY AND PRESENTING COMPLAINTS AT FOLLOW-UP

B. was seen for follow-up at the age of 7 years, 4 months. At follow-up, B. was just beginning first grade in a special class for language-disordered children. During the interval between the initial and follow-up evaluations, B. had received biweekly speech–language therapy in private sessions and had continued in his nursery school placement. At age 6, he had attended a regular Kindergarten class, where he lagged somewhat behind the other children in learning, although he seemed to get along well with his classmates. No other environmental changes had occurred.

B.'s mother described him as an active child who enjoyed playing soccer and riding his bike. The mother stated that, although he got along well with his peers in school and wanted to have friends, he did not see other children outside of school. Most of his time away from school was spent playing computer games, building cities with his Leggo set, and playing imaginary games with his Hot Wheels. He also helped around the house doing things such as putting away toys and clothes.

The mother stated that there was no problems in the home, and the major problem at school was difficulty remembering directions. Although there was no longer any marked distress at going to school, B. still showed some anxiety at being left by the parents.

The teacher reported that B. had a pleasant disposition, and was cooperative and eager to learn. She noted, though, that B. did have trouble understanding, was easily distracted, expressed more worries and fears than she felt appropriate, and often appeared to be in a world of his own.

B. was a cooperative, polite, and well-motivated boy during testing. He showed no apprehension about testing, and was comfortable about leaving his mother after ascertaining where she would be waiting for him. During informal conversation, B. was polite, but clearly preferred not to talk. His responses were typically brief, and frequently he used gestures as responses.

B.'s formal test results are shown in Table 5.1. In addition to the tests listed in the table, the GFTA was administered; some of B.'s misarticulations are given below.

Words misarticulated	*Articulations*
house	houth
pencil	penthil
sock	thock
mother	mudder

Table 5-1. B.'s Formal Test Results at Follow-Up

Test	Score (age or grade level)
Wide Range Achievement Test	
Reading	Nursery, ninth month
Arithmetic	Kindergarten, second month
Spelling	Kindergarten, entry
WISC-R (performance IQ)	
ITPA	
Auditory reception	5 years, 6 months
Visual reception	7 years, 0 months
Auditory association	4 years, 6 months
Visual association	6 years, 9 months
Grammatical closure	4 years, 6 months
Verbal expression	4 years, 10 months
Auditory memory	4 years, 3 months
Visual memory	6 years, 11 months
PPVT	5 years, 6 months
TACL	4 years, 4 months
Memory for Sentences Test (Spencer, 1958)	4 years
TOLD	
Oral vocabulary	5 years, 5 months
Grammatic completion	Below 4 years

car	ca
rabbit	wabbit
carrot	cawot

Some of B.'s responses during testing were as follows:

EXAMINER: Name three animals.
B.: Corky, Sam, Caesar. [These were his two cats and his dog.]
EXAMINER: Are those your pets?
B.: That be right.
EXAMINER: Can you name any other animals?
B.: No. Why you no got your shoes on?
EXAMINER: What's a shoe?
B.: My dad wear white shoes. In liquor stores.
EXAMINER: What's a horse?
B.: He eat grass.
EXAMINER: What's a cup?
B.: Drink. Water.
EXAMINER: What's a dress?
B.: Pink. My mama blue pants.
EXAMINER: What are stamps for?
B.: In the letter.
EXAMINER: What's a bird?
B.: Birds just fly away. Wake people up. Where you got this typewriter? (*gestures to tape recorder*)
EXAMINER: Can you tell me what you eat for breakfast?
B.: Cereal and sugar and . . . I got a bed in my room.

B. made these responses during a sentence imitation task:

EXAMINER: (Reading stimulus sentences) Mama is in the car.
B.: My mom in the car.
EXAMINER: We are going to buy some candy.
B.: Me go buy the candy.
EXAMINER: Jane wants to build a big castle in her playhouse.
B.: Playhouse, castle, big castle.
EXAMINER: Tom has lots of fun playing ball with his sister.
B.: Tom playing ball his sister.
EXAMINER: Mama asked Nancy to bring the brown dog into the house.

B.: In the house. don't let the dog out.

EXAMINER: Mama bought Susie a chocolate ice cream cone after the movie yesterday.

B.: Mommy bought a ice cream in the picture.

DISCUSSION

As is typical of children with developmental language disorder, even after a course of speech–language therapy, B. still showed marked receptive and expressive language difficulties at follow-up. The sample of responses from testing showed that B. had both grammatical and word-finding errors, and his sentence length was still much reduced from what would be expected for a child his age. His speech articulation was still below chronological age level, but less so than his expressive language skills. As is typical of many children with developmental language disorder, B.'s achievement test results at the beginning of first grade did not yet show marked learning impairments.

B.'s testing behavior was cooperative, but his concentration and attention span were limited. This is not unusual for children with developmental language disorder, even when the diagnostic criteria for attention deficit disorder are not met. Some of B.'s responses during testing were idiosyncratic, irrelevant, or perseverative; again, this is not unexpected for a child of his age with developmental receptive language disorder.

B. no longer demonstrated marked separation anxiety at follow-up. In particular, there were no instances of school refusal. There was some distress on separation from the parents, and there were some generalized anxiety symptoms; however, these were not causing a significant degree of functional impairment.

Case Illustration: "S."

Presenting Complaints and History

S. was initially seen at age 4 years, 3 months, when he was referred to a speech and language center by his pediatrician because he had not been communicating and had only acquired a few words. The speech pathologist assigned to work with S. requested psychiatric referral, complaining that S. was "weird" and unlike any other child she had ever treated. Prior to S.'s initial appointment, the speech pathologist telephoned to caution that S. was "untestable" and would have "unbelievable tantrums" if any demands were placed on him.

S.'s parents had major complaints regarding both S.'s speech and language development and his behavior. With regard to behavior, the parents were concerned about his decreased tolerance for frustration. They had noted problems with activity level, excitability, distractibility, delayed echolalia, daydreaming, and inability to stop repetitive activities (e.g., counting things, putting things in rows, flapping arms, and twisting fingers). These behaviors were sufficiently severe that the parents were unable to take S. out in public or to keep him in nursery school.

S. was the product of a cesarean delivery done under general anesthesia when his head wouldn't drop after 10 hours of labor. The medical history was unremarkable, except for allergy to milk as an infant and one episode of influenza at age 3½. The mother described S. as a friendly, affectionate baby who liked attention and had been no problem at all until age 3.

S.'s developmental milestones were as follows: smiling at parents at 3 months, turning over at 3 months, sitting at 8 months, crawling at 10 months, walking with help at 11 months, walking alone at 20 months, feeding himself at 24 months, weaning from bottle at 26 months, bowel-trained at 5 years, and dressing himself at 5 years.

The parents reported that S. had "always" been abnormal in speech and language development. He had not babbled as an infant, and had not said his first word until the age of 2. By the age of 3, S. had a vocabulary of 10 words he was using regularly, but by the age of 4, there had been little increase in language development. The statement "cup of juice" was the closest thing to a sentence he had used.

Overall Approach to the Evaluation

Although it was clear from the history that S. had some type of speech–language disorder, it was also clear that there was little hope of obtaining detailed testing information. The goals of the evaluation, then, were to attempt to determine the gross extent of verbal deficits, to establish whether there was a clear verbal–nonverbal discrepancy, and to see whether the verbal deficits were uniform across different areas of functioning. It was hoped that an informal testing approach would provide this information.

Clearly, there were major problems with S.'s behavior. He presented with a very complex picture in which the differential diagnosis had to consider mental retardation, infantile autism or other pervasive developmental disorder, attention deficit disorder, and obsessive–compulsive disorder.

Evaluation of S.'s behavior problems required an interview with the parents, covering a detailed history of S.'s social interactions (including differentiations between people, selective attachments, social overtures, social responses, and social play); the play history (including cognitive levels, content, type, and quality of play); and past and current psychiatric symptomatology. The latter were probed using the DICA parent interview (see Chapter 4, p. 114) and parent behavioral rating scales.

Because of S.'s language difficulty and his youth, the DICA child interview could not be used. However, S. was observed in play, unstructured, structured, and task-oriented situations in several sessions. Family interactions and interactions in the clinical setting were observed, although no information was obtained on peer interactions, since S. was not in school at the time of evaluation and had no playmates.

Procedures Selected and Data Collected

Due to S.'s lack of cooperation and attention, adequate formal testing could not be done. S. seemed to enjoy informal play, however, and was quite willing to look at books when they contained large, simple pictures. When multiple pictures were presented for language testing (as in the PPVT), S. began leaving his chair, screaming, laughing, and going rigid. Particularly disturbing was S.'s screaming, which was abnormally high in pitch and very loud.

During articulation testing with single pictures, S. was somewhat distracted and kept looking at himself in the mirror, but he did respond to questions, using words appropriately and spontaneously. His expressive language was essentially at the one-word stage, although there were some two-word utterances. He correctly labeled "car," "book," "bird," "drink," "flower," and "tree." He had a moderate degree of articulation impairment, with most medial and final consonants in words being omitted. He did not use any unusual or stereotyped expressions, but did have echolalia, tending to echo the other speaker rather than echoing his own speech. He used gestures and pointed to things he wanted.

Discussion and Differential Diagnosis

Possible differential diagnoses of S.'s behavior disorder included mental retardation, infantile autism, pervasive developmental disorder, obsessive–compulsive disorder, and attention deficit disorder. In both unstructured and structured settings, S. had significant problems with attention, impulsivity, and motor activity. He was more hyperactive and inattentive, as observed during language testing, when multiple stimuli were presented, but he was able to attend to other stimuli for longer periods of time. This suggested that the attentional difficulties were, to some degree, task-dependent.

The history from the parents of no significant problems (other than speech and language difficulty) prior to the age of 3; their account of S.'s being an affectionate baby; and the use of gestures as well as the relatedness observed by the speech-language examiner and the psychiatric examiner all suggested that a diagnosis of infantile autism was not appropriate. Although no formal IQ testing could be done, the history of normal developmental milestones did not suggest a diagnosis of general mental retardation. It was not possible to evaluate obsessional thinking; however, S. did not seem to have a true compulsion, but only rather repetitive, persistent behaviors.

A general approach to differential diagnosis of problems like those of S. is first to determine intellectual level; then to determine the level of language development; and then to consider whether the behavior is appropriate for chronological age, mental age, and language age. History and informal assessment suggested that S. was of normal intellectual potential. His language development was clearly abnormal; his behavior was clearly inappropriate for his chronological age and mental age, and also for his language age. Here the differential diagnosis hinged on S.'s social interaction, pattern of language deficits, play, and other behaviors.

Since there was a period of normal development, the diagnosis of infantile autism was not appropriate, but the diagnosis of pervasive developmental disorder was still possible. There was no suggestion that S. was presenting with an early form of schizophrenia, and since there was no history of organic insult or other relevant medical conditions, acquired aphasia with seizure disorder and disintegrative psychosis were also unlikely. Also, there was no history of parental neglect or abuse or of severe psychological deprivation; hence the possibility of some type of abnormal bonding pattern secondary to parental neglect and abuse was not appropriate.

It is clear that, in addition to the behaviors suggesting pervasive developmental disorder, there were also behaviors suggesting attention deficit disorder. However, a diagnosis of attention deficit disorder did not explain all of the behaviors presented by S. Thus, on the basis of the initial differential diagnosis, the most likely diagnoses were pervasive developmental disorder and attention deficit disorder. There are some clinicians who would not make the second diagnosis in the presence of the first.

Follow-Up Evaluation

INTERVAL HISTORY AND PRESENTING COMPLAINTS

S. was seen for follow-up evaluation approximately 4 years later, at the chronological age of 7 years, 3 months. In the interval since his first evaluation, he had been receiving speech therapy three times a week, had been working weekly with a social worker on his behaviors, and had been enrolled in nursery school and then kindergarten.

The parents reported that, although there had been considerable progress in speech and language, there were still many behavioral problems. These included (1) attention deficit symptoms (not being able to concentrate or pay attention for long; daydreaming; being restless and unable to sit still; acting as if driven by a motor; being easily frustrated; insisting his demands must be met; being irritable and quick to fly off the handle; being impulsive and acting without thinking); (2) conduct disorder symptoms (not feeling guilty after misbehaving; being cruel and bullying other children, not getting along with other children; being disobedient at home and at school; swearing or using obscene language; being cruel to animals; arguing; threatening people; talking back or being sassy); and (3) anxiety symptoms (fearing certain animals, situations, and places; whining; being withdrawn or not involved with others; worrying; being too fearful or anxious; crying a lot; and feeling worthless and inferior).

In addition, there were many other abnormal behaviors, including acting too young for his age; being confused or in a fog; getting hurt a lot or being accident-prone; being nervous, high-strung, or tense; not being liked by other children; being poorly coordinated or clumsy; repeating certain acts over and over; being secretive, showing off excessively or clowning; being stubborn, sullen, or irritable; screaming a lot; staring blankly; having sudden changes in mood or feelings; having temper tantrums; and showing strange behaviors.

S.'s school teacher described him as having tantrums and unpredictable behavior, showing low frustration tolerance, exhibiting drastic mood changes, and being too excitable and impulsive. She reported that learning, work habits, behavior, mood, and group participation were serious problems.

TESTING AT FOLLOW-UP

S.'s behavior at follow-up, although still characterized by periods of inattentiveness, extreme "silliness," and lack of motivation, was now adequate to permit us to obtain achievement and intelligence scores. The test scores obtained are presented in Table 5-2.

S.'s most striking linguistic feature was the inappropriateness of his responses to questions, which was responsible for

Table 5-2. S.'s Formal Test Results at Follow-Up

Test	Score (age or grade level)
Wide Range Achievement Test	
Reading of words	Third grade, first month
Arithmetic	Second grade, third month
Spelling	Second grade, second month
Gray Oral Reading Test	First grade, sixth month
WISC-R (performance IQ)	90
DASE	6 years
PPVT	5 years, 5 months
TACL	5 years, 2 months
Memory for Sentences Test	5 years, 0 months
Georgetown Language Screening Test	
Expressive language	Below 4 years

his low expressive language score. Even relatively simple questions such as "What is your name?" and "How many eyes do you have?" received inappropriate responses such as "I'm S. and I'm Spidey," and "Two take away one." In addition, other features of abnormal language use, such as echolalia, idiomatic word usage, and jargon, were observed. Below is a sample of S.'s language taken at follow-up.

EXAMINER: S., are you going to say "hi" to me?
S.: I got some—I got nice hair. I got cut hair.
EXAMINER: Would you say hello?
S.: Hi.
EXAMINER: Well, now tell me your name.
S.: I'm S. and I'm Spidey.
EXAMINER: Tell me about this picture.
S.: A little boy.
EXAMINER: Yes, a little boy. And what is he doing?
S.: He's sitting on a stool. Oh, there's a bear.
EXAMINER: Is that a bear? No, that's a pig. What's the pig doing?
S.: Oink, oink, oink.
EXAMINER: O.K. What's he doing?
S.: He's sitting down. A cake.

EXAMINER: Tell me about this one.
S.: A bike.
EXAMINER: It's not a bike. Look again (*picture shows a boy on a dog*).
S.: A kid.
EXAMINER: What's the boy doing?
S.: A dog.
EXAMINER: What's the boy doing to the dog?
S.: Petting. I hear the fire.
EXAMINER: What's the boy doing?
S.: He's sitting on the dog.
EXAMINER: Do you have any books at your school?
S.: Yup, but do you know what I have? I have a vator place.
EXAMINER: Tell me some more about your school.
S.: My school is my too many problems. I don't need the stuff they do. That's what I . . . Every time I get something to play, you know what happens?
EXAMINER: What?
S.: I do things that wrongs.
EXAMINER: You do things wrong? O.K. Now I want you to read a story in my book, S.
S.: (*Looking at book, page number "A-1"*)A four and a five, six four and six five and six.
EXAMINER: No, what's the first word?
S.: Wolfman, wolfman, wolfman.
EXAMINER: Stop being silly, S.
S.: (*Reads*) "Look, mother, look"—woo! (*Screams, then continues reading, choking at the end of each sentence*) "Look, mother, look (*choke*). I can go (*choke*). I go up (*choke*). I go down (*choke*). Come and play with me (*choke*)."
EXAMINER: That's very good reading, but why did you cough like that?
S.: I make extermation points.
EXAMINER: It sounded to me like you were coughing.
S.: I burp extermation points. What's that story called again?
EXAMINER: Let's talk a little about it, O.K.? What did the girl do in the story?
S.: She was like a wolflady and she's bad.
EXAMINER: Who was she talking to?
S.: Untrue. That's untrue.
EXAMINER: What did the girl ask her mother to do?

S.: Untrue. That's untrue. True.
EXAMINER: Do you want to read the next story?
S.: I don't wanna read. Not read too much.
EXAMINER: O.K., let's talk for a while.
S.: I got a 3 for reading or a 2 for reading? How about for nap? Gimme nap. Gimme—do my homework for me. (*Giggles*) Twenty-twenty.
EXAMINER: Stop being silly.
S.: I like to say twenty.
EXAMINER: What do you like to eat?
S.: Dragon.
EXAMINER: You're being awfully silly today, S.
S.: Because I like to eat dragon.

DISCUSSION

Although S. showed marked improvement in speech and language from the initial evaluation, he was still behind in all areas. Articulation (in which S. scored at the 6-year level) was not considered to be a real problem, but speech was still abnormal, characterized by both lack of intonation patterns and deviant overall pitch. Language skills were more impaired; vocabulary, language comprehension, language expression, auditory memory, and use of language were all problem areas.

S.'s language sample was, in many ways, characteristic of the language of a child who has pervasive developmental disorder. It could be seen that, although S. could form longer, grammatical sentences, he seemed to prefer shorter ones. In addition, S. had difficulty producing the correct names for objects, used neologisms, showed idiosyncratic word usage, and frequently gave responses that were inappropriate.

At the time of follow-up, the course of S.'s behavior development was most characteristic of the diagnosis of childhood-onset pervasive developmental disorder. Among the types of symptomatology present were perseverative acts, symptoms of attention deficit disorder, conduct disorder symptoms, and anxiety symptoms. Multiple diagnoses of attention deficit disorder, conduct disorder, and generalized anxiety disorder, would, however, not cover the panoply of these and of other abnormal behaviors, including secretive behavior, multiple and sudden changes in mood and feelings, and the other strange behaviors. Thus, the diagnosis of pervasive developmental disorder was most appropriate at the time of follow-up.

Like the treatment of infantile autism, the treatment of pervasive developmental disorder must be multipronged. Its goals must include fostering normal development in the cognitive, language, and social areas; promoting learning; reducing rigidity and stereotypic behavior; alleviating nonspecific maladaptive behaviors; and alleviating family distress.

CHAPTER 6

Educational and Psychiatric Effects of Developmental Language or Articulation Disorders

Educational Effects

Introduction and Definitions

This section concerns the relationship between developmental language or articulation disorders and learning disorders in children.

The definition of "learning disorders" is pivotal to both clinical practice and research, since prevalence rates, sample selection for research studies, and inclusion criteria for special education programs all depend on the definition used. In this work, we use the term "ability" to connote an underlying, often inferred, capacity; "performance" to describe an observed behavior; "deficit" to describe functioning at a level below that expected; and "disorder" to describe a recurring pattern causing distress, disability, or disadvantage to the individual. Thus, a "performance deficit" is functioning below expected levels that may suggest the presence of an "ability deficit" or disability.

Public Law 94-142 (1975) (the public school definition of learning disorder) and DSM-III provide two competing definitions of "learning disorder." The public school definition states that learning-disordered children are "those children who have a disorder in one or more of the basic psychological processes involved in understanding or in using language, spoken or written, which disorder may manifest itself in an imperfect ability to listen, think, speak, read, write, spell, or do mathematical calculations" (Sec. 602, ¶15). Excluded in this definition are "children who have learning problems which are primarily the result of visual, hearing, or motor handicaps; mental retardation; emotional disturbance; or environmental, cultural, or economic disadvantage" (Sec. 602, ¶15).

As Barkley (1981) points out, there are some problems with the U.S. Public Law 94-142 definition—namely, it does not stipulate the amount of performance deficit that constitutes a "disorder"; provide a reference standard such as age, IQ, or grade level; or define cognitive skills. Furthermore, its exclusion criteria are relatively loose, leaving unclear how educational or cultural deprivation may be involved or defined.

Unlike the public school definition of learning disorders, DSM-III does not stress underlying psychological processes. The DSM-III diagnosis of an academic skills disorder is determined by objective standardized measures of performance demonstrating skill levels below those expected, given the individual's schooling, chronological age, and mental age as derived by an individually administered IQ test. A more complete discussion of the issue of the definition and quantification of learning disorders can be found elsewhere (Barkley, 1981; Forness & Kavale, 1983a, 1983b; Schere, Richardson, & Bialer, 1980).

Types of Learning Disorders

Keogh, Major-Kingsley, Omori-Gordon, and Reid (1982) and Satz and Morris (1981) review in detail the controversy surrounding the classification of learning disorders. We concern ourselves here with the three subtypes of academic skills disorders specified in DSM-III: those involving reading, arithmetic, and written expression.

READING DISORDER

Barkley (1981) and Boder (1973) propose that there are three subgroups of developmental reading disorder, involving underlying disorders in language skills, sequencing and verbal expression, and visual and spatial skills. According to Barkley (1981), approximately 60% of all reading-disordered children have disordered language skills manifested in a verbal–performance discrepancy on IQ scores; mispronunciations in oral reading, supposedly due to association errors; and poor scores on tests of auditory discrimination or word finding. This group of disabled readers frequently has an early history of delayed language development and may be labeled "dysphonetic."

The subgroup of children who have underlying disorders of sequencing and verbal expression may comprise 10% to 20% of all children with developmental reading disorders (Barkley, 1981). These children, labeled by Boder (1973) "mixed dysphonetic," do poorly on all achievement tests; show little discrepancy between verbal and nonverbal IQ scores; and show poor articulation, handwriting, and recall of sentences.

The smallest subgroup of children with developmental reading disorders, according to Barkley (1981), are the 5% to 10% who do very poorly on tests of visual–spatial construction, drawing, and copying, and frequently score low on IQ performance subtests. These children, labeled "dyseidetic" by Boder (1973), are poor sight readers of words, even when dealing with simple, frequently encountered words. Spelling errors are usually phonetically correct, but often inaccurate in the letters used for a particular word. Unlike children with disordered language skills, these children do not make wild guesses at spelling. The use of good phonetic and analytic skills often enables those with disordered visual and spatial skills to progress through the early grades without detection.

ARITHMETIC DISORDER

Compared to the voluminous literature on developmental reading disorder, the literature on developmental arithmetic disorder is relatively sparse. Elsewhere (Baker & Cantwell, 1984a), we provide a detailed review of the literature.

Many experts believe that there are several subtypes of developmental arithmetic disorder. Multiple skills may be impaired in children with developmental arithmetic disorder. Auditory-verbal, visual-spatial, motor, memory, and attention deficits are often present.

The inability to comprehend or name mathematical terms and operations; failure to decode written problems into mathematical symbols; and inability to grasp concepts such as "more-less," "first-last," and "before-after" demonstrate the overlap of language skill deficits in both developmental arithmetic and developmental reading disorders. Hence, children with poor reading skills may manifest impairment when mathematics is taught through reading-based instructional methods (Kinsbourne & Caplan, 1979).

DISORDERS OF WRITTEN EXPRESSION

The literature on disorders of written expression, "specific spelling disorder," or "dysgraphia" is negligible. Barkley (1981) suggests that this disorder takes three forms: one with associated deficits in language development (especially the development of phonetic analytic skills); one with associated deficits in visual skills; and one with no apparent underlying deficits.

Spelling difficulties are rarely found in isolation from other learning difficulties; they usually occur together with reading difficulties or arithmetic difficulties. In "pure" dysgraphic children, the underlying problem may be a type of apraxia in the planning and execution of voluntary motor movements, particularly writing. These children do poorly on intelligence subtests (such as the WISC-R coding subtest) that require handwriting. It is often not until the late elementary or junior high school period that dysgraphic children come to professional attention; prior to this, written expression plays only a minor role in academic success.

Conclusions

This brief summary of the literature on learning disabilities leads to the following conclusions: "Learning-disordered children" cannot be considered a homogeneous subgroup. Most suffer from concurrent disorders of reading, spelling, and arithmetic. The overlap of deficits in language and visual-spatial skills renders "pure" learning disorders unlikely. Early communication disorders are likely precursors to developmental learning disorders.

Learning Disorders in Clinical Follow-Up Studies

The relationship between communication and learning disorders has been examined by true prospective studies, retrospective studies, and "catch-up" prospective studies. In the true prospective studies, children with communication disorders are followed over time for the development of learning disorders; in retrospective studies, the backgrounds of children with learning disorders are examined for any history of communication disorders; and in "catch-up" prospective studies, children with communication disorders are diagnosed by earlier records.

Table 6-1 summarizes published follow-up studies on children with communication disorders and the educational difficulties that they experience. Single case histories and samples that include fewer than eight children have not been included in the table. Sample sizes, study designs, and methods used vary greatly in these studies. However, the literature suggests that children with communication disorders are at risk for learning disorders; furthermore, children with language involvement are at greater risk for later learning disorders than children with speech involvement such as developmental articulation disorder. Reading difficulties are more severely affected than arithmetic skills.

Our study (described in more detail in the next section) found children from a community speech and hearing clinic to be at risk for developmental learning disorders. Follow-up revealed that the prevalence of developmental learning disorders increased over time, independent of intervention with speech and language therapy. In addition, there was a strong correlation between the presence of a developmental learning disorder and a psychiatric disorder, particularly attention deficit disorder, in these children. Thus, learning problems may affect communication disorders, psychiatric disorders, or both. Previous studies indicate that children without communication disorders who have attention deficit disorder are indeed at risk for developmental learning disorders. More research is greatly needed to identify those children (among the population of children with communication disorders) most at risk for the development of learning disorders; types of developmental learning disorders most likely to be manifested; and factors that increase the risk of developmental learning disorders.

Psychiatric Effects

It has been long recognized that children with communication disorders are at risk for various types of learning disorders. Not as well documented is the concurrent risk for psychiatric disorder. Elsewhere (Cantwell & Baker, 1977), we review literature dealing with the social, emotional, and behavioral outcome of children with various types of communication disorders, including stutterers and those with voice disorders, articulation problems, cleft palate, and language disorders. This review suggests that children with various types of communication disorders, considered as a group, do have an increased rate of psychiatric disorders, compared to peers with no communication disorders. Most at risk are those with global and receptive language disorders; children with pure speech or expressive language disorders are less likely to develop psychiatric problems. Duration, severity, and type of communication disorder may be correlated with type of psychiatric disorder. For example, children with a severe receptive language disorder often demonstrate a syndrome analogous to infantile autism early in their development.

Unfortunately, much of the literature in this area suffers from a lack of objective methods and operational diagnostic criteria for psychiatric disorder; confounding of the psychiatric and communication disorder variables; lack of operational

Table 6-1. Summary of Studies of Educational Outcome for Children with Speech/Language Disorders

	Research Sample		Follow-up		Speech/Language		Psychiatric	
Author(s)	Initial Size & Source	Ages	Number (%)	Ages	Methodology	Outcome	Methodology	Outcome
Aram and Nation (1980)	513 from speech clinic	Mean = 32 mo	63 (= 12%)	Mean = 95 mo	Parent, teacher questionnaires	40% with speech or language problems	Teacher questionnaire	40% with reading or spelling problems, 20% with math problems
Aram, Ekelman, and Nation (1984)	47 from speech clinic	3–7 yr	20 (= 43%)	13–17 yr	PPVT, TOAL, Goldman-Fristoe-Woodcock Auditory Selective Attention Test	19 or 20 had deficits on TOAL; 90% were below the 21st percentile on Goldman-Fristoe-Woodcock	Wide Range Achievement Test	Over 80% below the 25th percentile on the Wide Range Achievement Test
Cooper, Moodley & Reynell (1979)	119 from speech clinic	Range = 2–4 yr	38 (= 32%)	Range 7–10.5 yr	Teacher reports	80% "progressing"	Teacher reports	70% "making good progress"
deAjuriaguerra *et al.* (1976)	40	Range = 4.3–10.10 yr	17 (= 43%)	Range = 7.2–12.9 yr	Nonstandardized tests of speech and language	100% still dysphasic	WISC-R, classroom placement	14 of 17 had "scholastic problems"
Fundudis, Kolvin, and Garside (1980)	133 from epidemiologic sample	3 yr	102 (= 77%)	7 yr	ITPA, English Picture Vocabulary Test,[a] free speech sample analysis	100% still significantly impaired in speech or language	WISC, reading quotient, class placement, teacher reports	Average reading quotient = 80; 19 of 83 in special schools
M. Garvey and Gordon (1973)	retrospective follow-up	?[a]	53 from special school	Range = 4–14 yr	PPVT, free speech sample	37 of 58 requiring speech therapy	Teacher reports, class placement	Majority of cases in special schools; reading problems common

C. Griffiths (1969)	55 from special school	Range = 1–3 yr younger than follow-up ages	49 (= 89%)	Range = 7.5–16.5 yr	PPVT, Sentence repetition, ITPA, articulation test	45% below average in language; 43% defective in articulation	Shonell reading and spelling tests, teacher reports	75% in special classes or schools
Hall and Tomblin (1978)	retrospective follow-up	Mean = 6 yr	36 from speech clinic	Mean = 22 yr	Parent questionnaire	Language group: 50% still had a problem; articulation group: 5% (1 case) still had a problem	School records of Iowa Test of Basic Skills, Iowa Test of Educational Development if available	Language group: lower achievement score, reading worst problem; articulation group: no significant low scores
King, Jones, and Lasky (1982)	150 from speech clinic	3–6 yr	50 (= 33%)	13–20 yr	Interview with mother	42% with some type of speech/language problem	Interview with mother	52% with academic difficulties
Klackenberg (1980)	63 from epidemiological sample of 212	3 yr	Approximately 80%	20 yr	none	No information	School level at age 20	Speech delayed group scored below matched group of normals
Petrie (1975)	11 from special residential school	Range = 4–6 yr		18 mo later	Reynell Scales; ITPA; ratings of auditory discrimination	Very little progress; auditory memory had least progress	Southgate Reading Test	All children could recognize some words
Sheridan and Peckham (1975, 1978)	212 from special school	7 yr	First Follow-up = 190 (90%) Second Follow-up = 180 (= 85%)	First Follow-up = 11 yr Second Follow-up = 16 yr	Parent and teacher reports	44% had satisfactory speech at 11 yr; 49% had satisfactory speech at 16 yr	Type of school, school reports	65% in regular school at 11 yr; 70% in regular school at 16 yr
Wolpaw, Nation, and Aram (1979)	47 from speech clinic	Mean = 4.8 yr	30 (= 64%)	Mean = 9.4 yr	PPVT, NSST, nonstandardized articulation and repetition tasks	One group of cases showed no change; other group had various changes	Class placement	7 children were EMR in classes for the educable mentally retarded; 13 in classes for the learning disabled

[a]Brimer & Dunn 1962.
[b]A question mark (?) indicates that no information was provided.

diagnostic criteria for both the presence and type of communication disorder; use of unrepresentative samples for study (e.g., use of children with communication disorders who have been referred to a psychiatric facility); and lack of appropriate control groups.

Our ongoing study of 600 first referrals to a community speech and hearing center disclosed 352 children with a disorder involving both speech and language, 45 children with a disorder involving language only, and 203 children with a speech disorder but normal language. They ranged in age from 2 to 16 years, with a mean age of 5 years, 10 months; 60% were under 6 years of age, 32% were between 6 and 11.9 years of age, and 8% were 12 years of age or above. Males constituted 69% of the sample, an age and sex distribution representative of first referrals to a large community speech and hearing center. The distribution of social classes and ethnic groups was not significantly different from that of the greater Los Angeles/San Fernando Valley, California, region from which the sample was drawn. To our knowledge, this is the first study using a large, psychiatrically unselected sample of children with a variety of communication disorders, employing rigorous psychiatric methodology. The methodology and results from this study have been reported in several publications (Baker & Cantwell, 1982, 1984a, 1985, in press-a, in press-b; Cantwell & Baker, 1980a, 1980b, 1983, 1985, in press).

Approximately one-half of the children in this study had some diagnosable DSM-III psychiatric disorder. About 25% had an overt behavior disorder (such as attention deficit disorder, oppositional disorder, or conduct disorder), and 20% had emotional disorders (such as one of the anxiety disorders). Mental retardation affected only 6% of the sample; developmental learning disorders affected 21% of the sample.

In addition to the high prevalence of psychiatric disorder in the group as a whole, it was found that children in the different groups of communication disorders had varying rates of psychiatric illness. Only 31% of the children with a pure speech disorder had a psychiatric disorder; for those with a speech and language disorder, the prevalence jumped to 58%; and in the pure language group it was 73%. Those children with receptive language disorders had significantly more psychiatric disorders than those with expressive disorders.

Children with at least one DSM-III Axis I diagnosis differed from children with no psychiatric diagnosis on a variety of factors, including type of communication disorder, level of language comprehension, level of language expression, performance intelligence, verbal intelligence, presence of language-processing problems, presence of developmental disorders, and presence of psychosocial stressors. Linguistic diagnoses were the most critical factors in distinguishing the psychiatrically ill from the psychiatrically well group.

These data suggest not only that children with communication disorders are at risk for the development of psychiatric disorders, but also that speech and language factors play a major role in both the prevalence and type of psychiatric disorder. Epidemiological studies suggest that these psychiatric findings are representative. Stevenson and Richman (1976) examined 700 3-year-old children in London and found that 24 had an expressive language delay. Of these language-delayed children, 59% had significant behavioral problems, compared to only 14% in the group who had no significant language delay. At a follow-up of this epidemiological sample at age 8 years (Stevenson, Richman, & Graham, 1985), it was found that those children who initially had lower abilities in language structure had significantly more behavioral deviance than those who initially had higher abilities in language structure.

In a similar epidemiological study, Fundudis, Kolvin, and Garside (1980) selected 133 children with significant language delay from a total population of 3300 3-year-olds in Newcastle, England. Compared to normal controls, those with a significant language delay had problems with attention span, self-confidence, sociability, liking school, motor activity, and rapport, and displayed more psychiatric disorders.

If children with communication disorders are at risk for the development of psychiatric disorder, does treatment of the speech and language disorder affect the psychiatric disorder? This remains an unanswered question. No published studies have concentrated on the psychiatric status over time of children with communication disorders. Limited information about psychiatric outcome can be elicited from brief comments

Table 6-2. Summary of Studies of Psychiatric Outcome for Children with Speech/Language Disorders

	Research Sample		Follow-up		Speech/Language		Psychiatric	
Author(s)	Initial Size & Source	Ages	Number	Ages	Methodology	Outcome	Methodology	Outcome
Aram, Ekelman, and Nation (1984)	47 from speech clinic	3–7 yr	20 (= 43%)	13–17 yr	PPVT, TOAL, Goldman-Fristoe-Woodcock Auditory Selective Attention Test	19 of 20 had some language deficits	Achenbach Teacher Questionnaire (for n = 17)	Significantly below norms in social competence measure
deAjuriaguerra *et al.* (1976)	40 from patient caseload	Range = 4.3–10.10 yr	17 (= 40%)	Range = 7.2–12.9	Nonstandardized tests of articulation, perception, synonyms, narration, comprehension	All still dysphasic; auditory-verbal perception almost unchanged	Behavioral observations	Diagnoses were: "normal" (5), "preneurotic" (7), "psychotic" (5)
Fundudis, Kolvin, and Garside (1980)	133 from epidemiological sample	3 yr	102 (= 77%)	7 yr	ITPA, EPVT, analyses of free speech sample	18 "deviant"; 84 "significantly impaired" in speech or language	Rutter Teacher and Parent Questionnaires, Junior Eysenck Personality Inventory, interview	18 "deviant" (with mental retardation or autism), rest had significantly more abnormal scores on all psychiatric measures
M. Garvey and Gordon (1973)	Retrospective follow-up	?[a]	53 from special school	Range = 4–14 yr	PPVT, analysis of spontaneous speech sample	37 of 58 needed speech therapy at follow-up	School reports	Persistent behavior problems noted

C. Griffiths (1969)	55 from special school	Range = 1–3 yr younger than follow-up ages	49 (= 89%)	Range = 7.5–16.5 yr	PPVT, sentence repeption, ITPA, articulation test	45% below average in language development, 43% had articulation defects	Parent, teacher ratings using nine 5-point scales	25% had poor social development, 45% had poor emotional development
Klackenberg (1980)	63 from epidemiological sample of 212	3 yr	Approximately 80%	20 yr	?	?	If "registered under Child Welfare Act" (minor offenses)	More minor offenses in speech delayed group than in Normals; 6 had been in a reformatory
Paul, Cohen, and Caparulo (1983)	14 "childhood aphasics" from psychiatric clinic	Range = 2–11 yr	11 (= 79%)	various	PPVT, Reynell, Sequenced Inventory of Communication Development, Receptive-Expressive-Emergent Language Scales	"Slight to moderate improvement	Review of chart notes	"Slight improvement" in "behavioral difficulties"
Petrie (1975)	11 from special residential school	Range = 4–6 yr	?	18 months later	Reynell Language Scales, ITPA, Auditory Discrimination Rating	Very little progress; auditory memory had least progress	Bristol Social Adjustment Scales	7 of 11 "unsettled"; all had signs of shyness or withdrawal
Sheridan and Peckham (1975, 1978)	212 from special school	7 yr	190 180 (= 85%)	First follow-up: 11 yr Second follow-up: 16 yr	Parent and teacher reports	Satisfactory speech in 44% at 11 years; in 49% at 16 years	Bristol Social Adjustment Scales	30% maladjusted at 11 years; (no information for age 16)

[a]A question mark (?) indicates that no information was provided.

found in some published follow-up studies of communication disorders. Table 6-2 contains a summary of follow-up studies with sample sizes of nine or more communication-disordered children. As with the studies in Table 6-1, sample sizes, sources of the samples, and psychiatric methodology vary greatly. Nevertheless, these data suggest that when these children are followed up over time, a substantial number do have significant degrees of psychopathology.

In our study, approximately 400 children have been followed up at the time of the present writing; almost 90% of these have had speech and language intervention. Very few have had any other types of intervention, especially psychiatric intervention. Four years after initial evaluation, a substantial number of these children have shown marked improvement in speech and language functioning, with 26% testing within normal limits. However, the prevalence rates of psychiatric disorders and of developmental learning disorders have actually increased, suggesting that speech and language intervention alone is inadequate to alleviate the psychiatric and developmental learning disorders that these children may develop. In our study, there is a correlation between development of a learning disorder and development of a psychiatric disorder; those children with developmental learning disorders have had higher rates of psychiatric disorder than children without learning disorders, both initially and at follow-up.

CHAPTER 7

Intervention Strategies for Developmental Language Disorder and Developmental Articulation Disorder

The Importance of Early Intervention

The discussion presented in Chapter 6 shows that children with developmental speech and language disorders are at risk for both psychiatric and educational problems, and that these problems appear to be long-standing. The majority of follow-up studies, including our own, suggest that these children may suffer a variety of continuing or residual problems in nonlinguistic areas long after the speech or language problems have been remediated.

Because of the long-standing nature of speech and language dysfunctions, and the associated problems that tend to develop for these children, we believe that it is critical that any intervention with these children be done as early as possible. Although the literature provides no definitive answers as to whether early intervention with speech and language prevents the development of associated psychiatric and educational problems, the literature does lead us to hypothesize that this might be the case. Therefore, it is prudent that speech and language intervention for these children be initiated prior to entering school. Since language development is most rapid at the preschool ages, children who are untreated during this period tend to fall more and more seriously behind their peers.

Ideally, all children who are behind in speech or language development should receive speech and language therapy. However, in cases where limited therapeutic facilities are available, and choices must be made as to which children can receive special attention, then therapeutic efforts should be concentrated on those children who are most at risk for the development of secondary problems and those who are most likely to benefit from treatment. Among the factors to be considered when referring a child for speech or language therapy are the significance of the child's problem; the appropriateness of the child's language with regard to other developmental milestones and the environment; and the probability of successful therapy, based on the child's motivation and behaviors. In general, those children with disorders of language comprehension, production, or processing should receive the highest priorities for receiving speech–language therapy, whereas children with problems limited to speech production should receive a lower priority for treatment.

Factors to Consider in a Treatment Program

Since most children with developmental language disorder need help not only in the linguistic area but also educationally and behaviorally, the question of priorities within treatment arises. Unfortunately, we are unaware of any research addressing itself to this issue. Although we recommend that the primary concentration of therapeutic effort be in the linguistic area, it is also important to remediate any etiological, medical, or environmental factors that could interfere with speech or language therapy. Such factors include severe attentional deficits or behavioral abnormalities, seizure disorders, hearing loss, or severe lack of environmental stimulation.

This chapter discusses the various types of speech–language, educational, and psychiatric interventions that may be used. In addition, there is a discussion of some exercises and games that parents can employ to help with speech or language development.

Parental Roles in Intervention for Developmental Language Disorder

In recent years, a number of speech and language pathologists have recommended that parents work at home with their language-impaired children to increase the children's language skills (Clements, Evans, Jones, Osborne, & Upton, 1982; Cooper & Griffiths, 1978; S. Davis & Marcus, 1980; McDade, 1981; Rondal, 1980; Spradlin & Siegal, 1982). The rationale behind these recommendations is that the speech therapy setting is an unnatural one, and thus skills learned in such a setting may not generalize to the total environment. Additional support for these recommendations comes from observations that the effectiveness of speech–language therapy seems to be highly correlated with the frequency of sessions.

The literature on normal child language acquisition provides some theoretical justification for parental involvement with language-disordered children. This literature suggests that in normal children the speed of speech and language acquisition is correlated with the amount and type of parental input the children receive (Cross, 1978; Nelson, 1973; Salzinger, Patenaude, & Lichtenstein, 1975; Todd & Palmer, 1968). This appears to be particularly significant in the early years of language acquisition.

Despite these findings, there is a need for caution before recommending active parental involvement with language treatment. The amount of parental involvement in taking a child to and from tutors and therapists and in trying to cope with behavior problems in the home may already be considerable. It is important that other aspects of family life not suffer as "all-out" parental attention is devoted to the language-delayed child. Furthermore, working with language delays is a tedious and complicated task, requiring skills and patience that frequently may only be found in a trained therapist. Shelton (1978) describes training parents to work with their disordered children in making certain auditory associations and discriminations. Even though the parents were instructed to accept any responses that the children produced, there were a number of instances of parents reporting frustration and anger at the children's repeatedly incorrect responses. Goda (1970) also discusses the dangers of parental involvement in speech remediation, noting that, for a parent, a teaching role is somewhat incompatible with a loving and supportive role.

Below, we provide a discussion of some techniques that parents can use when working with their language-disordered children. These techniques should be attempted only by those parents who are eager to work with their children, and such efforts should be maintained only so long as they can provide positive experiences for both parents and children.

Specific Techniques for Facilitating Language Development

Forming Meaningful Interactions

The literature on normal child language acquisition suggests that high-quality parental interactions are important for language development. Such interactions involve being with the child and talking to him, rather than attempting to "teach" him language. The content of what is said is important only in that the interactions are meaningful and of interest to the child. Hubbell (1977) stresses that "verbal interaction is more important than verbal stimulation" (p. #225). Eisenson and Ogilvie (1983) concur: "[F]or a language environment to be effective, it must impinge on the child and be meaningful. . . . Any meaningful communication with the child should aid speech development" (p. #202).

Thus, during interactions with the language-delayed child, it is not necessary for the parents to concern themselves with presenting examples of vocabulary or sentence structures. To the contrary, it may be best for the parents to try to simplify their speech and to simultaneously use gestures to communicate, in order to gear their speech down to the child's level of understanding. If the child's level of language is very low, it may be necessary for the parents to limit utterances to single-word "sentences" with pauses in between.

Below are some suggestions of specific ways to enrich parent–child interactions in order to facilitate language development. These suggestions are based on techniques that have been shown to be associated with more rapid or more advanced language acquisition in normal children. Readers interested in more detailed suggestions on how parents can work with children at home are referred to the following works: Becker (1971), Hubbell (1977), Rosner (1979), Schumaker and Sherman (1978), and Semel (1976).

Encouraging Speech and Teaching Words

Parents should talk as much as possible to their children (even to young babies) during routine activities such as bathing, dressing, and playing. Such interactions should be routine and natural, and should focus on people, objects, or events that are immediately present in the environment. For example, when dressing a young child, a parent can say something like "Here's your foot," "Here's your hand," and so on. With severely language-delayed children, the parents should try to use short sentences (one to four words) and to repeat the sentences often. There is no evidence that using a special set of simplified words ("beddie-bye," "bow-wow") or talking in a high-pitched tone of voice ("baby talk") is helpful to the child (DePaulo & Bonvillian, 1978), and hence these should be avoided.

For parents who are particularly eager to work with their nonverbal children, reading from nursery rhymes or children's books is the next step. Readings should occur for brief periods of time (under 15 minutes) each day, and should be done in a pleasant tone of voice, with slow, clear speech. Books should be chosen for large, colorful pictures, so that older children can "read" along by looking at the pictures. When interacting with a child in this way, the parent should give the child an opportunity to respond with sounds or spontaneous speech.

Books can also be used to develop a child's vocabulary. While looking at the books together, the parent can point to individual pictures and name the items. This procedure has been called "modeling," and has been shown to increase the child's use of language (Cazden, 1965; Odom, Liebert, & Hill, 1968). Modeling can be applied to sentence structures as well as single words (e.g., "There's the cat," "There's a boy jumping," "That girl is reading," "Here's a little dog," "Here's a big dog").

Of particular value is an individualized picture book made by cutting pictures out of magazines or taking photos of people or objects having personal significance. Appropriate objects for such a book are things that move or act on their own (e.g., people, pets, vehicles) and things upon which the child himself can act (e.g., toys, food, certain clothing like shoes).

The parent can teach additional words to the child by pointing out objects in the immediate environment and labeling them. The same label should be used consistently, since switching to different words will inevitably confuse the language-delayed child.

When the child begins to speak, his efforts should be rewarded with parental attention, smiles, praise, touching, and/or repeating what the child has said. Parental reinforcement of any type has been shown to have substantial effect on children's utterances, and multiple types of reinforcement have been shown to be more effective than any single type (Hursh & Sherman, 1973). Any meaningful and appropriate response from a child should, therefore, be rewarded. If the child spontaneously uses an incorrect label, he can gently be corrected in a positive way. Parents should avoid correcting the child's grammatical and articulation errors, however. It appears that for language-delayed children, a "correcting" approach of this type may actually inhibit language development and lessen the child's interest in communicating (Filer, 1981; Shelton, Arndt, & Miller, 1961).

As the child begins to speak, the parents can gradually increase the length of their own utterances and the variety of vocabulary items.

Increasing the Child's Utterance Length

For children who are producing single-word utterances, there are several techniques that can be employed to increase the utterance length. The first technique is called "expansion," and consists of immediately repeating back what the child has said, but adding something to the utterance. A number of studies have shown that frequent use of expansions (to approximately 30% of all utterances) by mothers is correlated with increases in spontaneous utterance length in children (Cazden, 1965; Cross, 1978; Feldman & Rodgon, 1970). Expansions can be relatively short utterances that are appropriate and relevant, such as the following: (child) "Car," (mother) "Yes, there's a car"; (child) "Play ball," (mother) "You want to play ball"; (child) "Cookie," (mother) "That's a big cookie"; (child) "Baby crying," (mother) "The baby is crying."

Two other techniques that parents can use to facilitate language usage in children are called "prompting" and "recasting." Prompting is simply asking questions of the child while supplying all or part of the sentence structure for the expected answer. Some examples of prompts include "It's not a bus, is it?" "The car is what color?" "What do we do with flowers? Flowers go in a. . . ." "You want to go where?" Studies suggest that prompting may be a less valuable technique than either modeling or expansion. However, parents may wish to increase the amount of prompting to provide variety in interactions.

Recasting is repeating the child's utterance back to him, but modifying its structure in some way. For example, the child's utterance can be modified by substituting a pronoun or synonym for the word(s) the child has used, changing verb tense, or adding other words to form a more adult-like utterance. Like expansions and prompts, recasting should be relevant to the environmental context to which the child is attending. Some examples of recasting are these: (child) "Billy's bad," (mother) "Yes, he's being naughty today"; (child) "Doggie likes bones," (mother) "Yes, the doggie did like the bones."

Semiformal Approaches to Facilitating Language Development

There are now several behavioral programs that use parents as the primary language therapists and emphasize work in the home (S. Davis & Marcus, 1980; Yule & Berger, 1972). While some authors have reported considerable success using parents as speech–language therapists, we have not ourselves seen such programs in effect. Caution is necessary before encouraging parents to work intensely with a child's language, since language therapy must be carefully geared to the developmental level of the child and must follow appropriate developmental steps. Furthermore, very intense parental involvement in language therapy can produce an unpleasant mood of work for the child and frustration for the parents. Nonetheless, if formulated as games, more structured interactions between parent and child do appear to be successful in increasing particular language skills. Some games and interactions are discussed below.

EXERCISES IN VOCABULARY AND CONCEPTS

At the simplest level, naming is a useful activity for building and strengthening vocabulary. A game can be constructed in which the child names everything the parent points to, and then point to things for the parent to name. Trips to zoos, parks, and other places are good settings for this game, although it can also be played around the house and yard. Variants of the game "Twenty Questions" are also valuable—the parent can be "thinking" of some object or activity and can provide progressive clues or can let the child ask questions to identify the object. The roles can then be reversed, with the child thinking of an object and the parent guessing.

For the younger child, imaginative games such as "store," "shopping," "school," packing for a trip," "building a house," and "doctor" can be used to encourage vocabulary usage and development.

More sophisticated vocabulary games for older children

include defining objects (e.g., "Tell me everything you can about a . . . "—encouraging use of words describing color, shape, function, location, taste, etc.); listing items in word classes (e.g., "How many animals [foods, kinds of cars, vegetables, games, trees, furniture, rooms in a house, sports, flowers, birds] can you name?"); having the child give the functions of objects instead of names of objects; and having the child answer riddles ("What do you wear on your head?", "What has sleeves?", or "What runs on electricity?").

EXERCISES IN AUDITORY COMPREHENSION AND AUDITORY ATTENTION

Exercises to improve comprehension of spoken language can also be formulated as games for the child. One such game is "Simon Says" (in which the child can learn to attend to commands of various lengths and complexities). "Find it" is another such game; using household objects, the child is asked first to find single-word items, then paired-word items ("boy walking," "pink coat," "six ducks"), and finally items described in longer phrases and sentences (e.g., "the big ball under the little chair").

For younger children, games involving listening for sounds can be helpful in developing auditory attention and discrimination skills. For example, one such game might involve having the child identify common sounds that he hears but cannot see being made (e.g., clapping, snapping fingers, knocking, opening and closing the door, etc.). Or the parent can say a list of words and have the child clap whenever he hears a particular word or type of word (e.g., the name of a color).

Older children can be told (or read) simple stories and asked questions about the content of the stories. The parent should start with short, single-sentence stories, and gradually increase the amount the child must decode before asking the questions.

EXERCISES IN AUDITORY DISCRIMINATION

Auditory discrimination can be practiced by having the parent say pairs of words for the child to identify as either the same or different. Obviously, in order to do this, the child must have already acquired the concepts of "same" and "different." The parent should begin with pairs of words that sound very different (e.g., "cat," "dog") and gradually reduce the differences, working toward pairs of words that differ in only one sound ("cat," "cap"). When doing this, the parent should be sure that he does not give away the difference by using a pattern of contrastive stress when he says the words.

It is helpful for the child with auditory discrimination problems to learn to use the sentence context to help discriminate words. A game of "silly or good" can be played, with the parent presenting sentences for the child to label as appropriate or inappropriate (e.g., "I hurt my back," "I hurt my black"). Another such task involves reading the child a story and occasionally saying a wrong word. The child must be alert to immediately identify and correct the wrong word.

EXERCISES IN VERBAL EXPRESSION

The parent can encourage the child's use of verbal language by questions that gradually increase in complexity. For example, the parent can begin with simple yes–no questions ("Can dogs fly?" "Do chairs eat?") and increase the difficulty to "what" or "when" questions ("What color is milk?" "What season is warmest?" "When do we sleep?") and finally to "why" questions ("Why does Daddy work?" "Why do people sleep?). Another technique is to read an incomplete sentence or story and have the child fill in the missing word or words.

EXERCISES IN AUDITORY MEMORY AND SEQUENCING

Practice in auditory memory involves repeating things ranging from single words to sentences to be recalled. For example, the parent can say a list of items to be repeated back, as in "I am going on a trip and taking in my suitcase a . . ."). Or the child can be asked to perform some task, such as arranging items in a certain way ("pencil under book," "pencil between book and crayon," "blue, then red, then green crayon"). The items presented should range from single words, to paired words, to longer word strings and sentences involving abstract items.

Recall of stories is an exercise that can be used to practice both auditory memory and verbal expression. The parent should tell or read a simple story of 2, 3, or 4 sentences and have the child retell the story as accurately as possible. A more complex variant of this task is the "reporter" game, in which the child listens to a story on the radio or television and "reports" it to the parent.

Speech and Language Therapy

Most speech and language pathologists agree that speech and language therapy is essential for children with developmental articulation or language disorders. Eisenson and Ogilvie (1983), for example, state, "There is little question that significant clinical language disorders are not reversible without intervention" (p. 201).

Despite this agreement on the importance of language intervention, there are few controlled studies assessing the outcome of various forms of speech and language intervention (Keely, Shemberg, & Carbonell, 1976; Muma & Pierce, 1981; Panagos & Griffith, 1981). The extent of observed improvement in children undergoing speech and language therapy that is due to normal maturation as opposed to intervention is not clearly known.

Currently, there are a variety of methods of language therapy available. The literature shows papers supporting and rejecting each of these methods; it simply is not known what is the best approach to language therapy. The psychiatrist needs only to be aware of the different types of therapy available, in order to propose an alternative method should it appear that the child is not progressing well. For this reason, we present below a brief outline of the various types of language therapy. The reader should keep in mind, however, that all forms of therapy do not fit clearly into the various schools of thought; many therapists use an eclectic approach. Furthermore, within the various schools of therapy, the use of differing procedures (such as structured activities, expansions, reinforcements, free play, or directed play) can occur.

General Principles

In order to provide some criteria by which particular therapies can be judged, we mention here some of the general principles that are largely agreed upon by various schools of thought.

Most speech–language pathologists concur that the primary aim is to develop language skills for social communication. Thus, the development of language skill takes precedence over refining speech articulation skills. For the severely apraxic child who cannot produce speech sounds, it may be most appropriate to begin with a gestural system of communication (Deuel, 1983). Mere parroting of words or sentences is insufficient; the child must be taught rules for generating his own sentences in appropriate situations.

Therapy should not be random but planned. Assessment of the child's current linguistic and nonlinguistic skills facilitates identification of the "next steps" to be acquired. Presentation of increasingly difficult tasks can then be employed to extend the child's skill level.

Generalization of skills learned in the therapy setting to the "real world" outside is essential. For this reason, some therapists suggest that the therapy setting be unstructured. Other therapists feel that structure is necessary for learning, and recommend using minor changes such as different activities or different seating to encourage generalization.

Therapy should be fun and rewarding. Usually verbal attention and responses from the therapist are sufficient rewards. But for young children (for whom verbal praise may be valueless or even frightening), rewards such as food items can be used. Verbal play can be encouraged to help avoid frustration.

Periodic re-evaluation of progress is necessary, with attention to the appropriate usage of language in the social context as well as to grammatical acquisition. Therapy goals must include eliminating persistent jargon, inappropriate remarks, or echoing. Polite phrases ("please," "thank you") and social "rules" (taking turns, listening before responding) are to be modeled.

The Cognitive-Developmental Approach

One method of language intervention is heavily influenced by Piaget's (1952) work suggesting that language development is based on the prior development of sensor-motor, conceptual, representational, and symbolic behaviors. The proponents of this approach stress cognitive skills, such as matching, discrimination, and categorization of objects. The basis of this method is the use of a structured program of semantic development, which begins by assessing the child's level of concepts and vocabulary, and then builds on this through the direct and immediate pairing of a word with a corresponding experience. Rather than being taught the prepositions "on," "over," and "under," the child might be taught awareness of sidedness, directionality, space, and distance in various types of functional situations. Once single lexical forms are established, the child is then taught two-word utterances that represent semantic relations of different kinds.

Recent variations of this approach are the so-called "neurolinguistic programs" (Bandler & Grinder, 1979) designed to cause neural reorganization of verbal processes. Farmer and Goldworthy (1982) and Fontana and Diaper (1981) have studied movement therapy and found it to have no effects on language development. The new neurolinguistic therapy has received no scientific study to support its claims.

The Auditory Processing Approach

Another method of language therapy involves working on auditory skills such as perception, discrimination, and memory. This method arises from work in the areas of perceptual psychology and speech perception and aims to identify, by tests such as the ITPA, the child's areas of greatest deficit. There is considerable controversy whether such training results in improvement of language development (Hammill & Larsen, 1974; Kavale, 1981; Semel & Wiig, 1981; Sowell, Parker, Poplin, & Larsen, 1979). Due to differing samples and procedures in evaluating such approaches, their effectiveness cannot be determined at present.

The Linguistic Approach

Within the linguistic model, intervention focuses on the grammatical structures that are absent or deviant in the language-disordered child. This approach generally views the language-disordered child as a "passive learner" who must be systematically taught structures, beginning with the simplest and progressing to the more difficult. A number of preplanned programs have been developed using stimulus–response techniques such as modeling and expansions. Generally, comprehension precedes production in intervention.

The Pragmatic Approach

The newest approach to language intervention is the "pragmatic" or "naturalistic" approach, based upon the belief that intervention must demonstrate to the child the functional benefit of communication. Pragmatic programs first teach those skills thought to precede language development (drawing attention to oneself, responding to social approaches, initiating social interaction, and using social agents to obtain ends). Then the semantic relations found in early language development are taught (agent + action and agent + object), and finally, a full range of pragmatic rules of language usage is taught (labeling, repeating, answering, requesting an action, requesting an answer, calling, greeting, and protesting).

This therapeutic approach tends to be unstructured; a variety of linguistic structures are presented simultaneously, and the child is treated in group or other "naturalistic" settings.

Educational Intervention

Most children with developmental language disorder suffer from learning problems. In general, those children with moderate or severe developmental language disorder need to be in either a special class or special school setting, where they can receive help in establishing peer relationships and appropriate behaviors, as well as in working toward speech, language, and educational achievement. Less severely language-impaired children may be able to remain in a regular classroom if they receive special attention or help. "Pull-out" help during regular classes may be valuable academically, but must be considered carefully in view of the disadvantages of stigmatizing the child as "different," disrupting the regular classroom, and limiting the amount of time the child receives with a specialist. After-school tutoring may be preferable, since it not only can provide academic assistance, but also can teach necessary study habits and techniques.

Educational Modifications in the Classroom

One of the major justifications for a special class is that the classroom can then be modified. For the child with problems in auditory discrimination, auditory memory, or language comprehension, a highly structured classroom setting with quiet, nondistracting surroundings is essential. It is also necessary for the teacher to make modifications in his speech to facilitate the language-disordered child's comprehension. The teacher may need to speak at a slower-than-normal rate, frequently repeat or reword utterances, supplement his talk with gestures and facial expressions, and eliminate figurative language or pronouns. In order to get and keep the child's attention, it may be necessary to touch him or to call his name periodically. When asking the child questions, the teacher may have to allow him more time to respond.

In the regular classroom setting, a child with developmental language disorder needs to be given special modifications. He should be seated as far away from distractions as possible and checked periodically to be sure he understands what is going on. It may be necessary to teach the child special techniques (e.g., visualizing, making drawings) for remembering oral instructions.

Children with developmental language disorder generally require special teaching approaches, such as the use of visual aids. In teaching spelling and reading, such methods as "color phonics," modified alphabets, or "process training" can be used, but recent studies suggest that the choice of method used may be less important than the manner in which the methods are applied (Zigmond, Vallecorsa, & Leinhardt, 1982). Teaching must be consistent and child–teacher interaction frequent.

Educational Modifications in the Home

There are a number of things parents can do to help a child educationally at home.

PROVIDE STRUCTURE

Just as the child with developmental language disorder needs structure in the classroom, he also needs structure at home. Parents should make an effort to keep activities at home as routine as possible, always informing the child in advance should there be any change. Large amounts of unstructured time are to be avoided. Consistency is important in disciplinary matters.

The language-disordered child should have his own nondistracting, quiet place to work or relax when he feels frustrated. When the child is approaching any task (meals, play, and especially homework), the area should be uncluttered. To facilitate structure, places for possessions should be designated and labeled.

Homework especially requires both organization and parental encouragement. The table or desk should be cleared of tempting unnecessary objects, and interruptions and distractions should be minimized. A study schedule should be set, and during study time the child should not be permitted to receive telephone calls. The parents should establish a routine by having the child spend regular time in the study area even if he has no homework. This avoids reinforcing not bringing work home. While it is not recommended for parents to sit with the child doing homework or to become overinvolved in the assignments, there are ways in which the parents can help with homework. For the language-disordered child who frequently has a short attention span, it is helpful to break up homework assignments into chunks short enough for the child to complete before his interest is lost. The parent might suggest, "Just do three problems now. Then you can play for 15 minutes. The you'll finish the last three problems." Thus parents can also check assignments at frequent intervals in order to catch errors before they become a long series of mistakes.

ENCOURAGE LEARNING

Parents should make every effort to encourage learning and to reward interest shown in learning; for instance, they should verbalize their own curiosity about words and share discoveries of how things work. The child needs to be given books of his own, and shown such study techniques as how to use a library, dictionary, or map. If the child has difficulty in reading but objects to "baby" books, he may feel important if asked to read these stories to younger children.

The language-disordered child can benefit from teamwork between his parents and his teacher. Parental rewards ranging from verbal praise to special trips can be used not only to encourage school work, but to encourage the reduction of negative behaviors that interfere with learning (e.g., daydreaming, disruptions, talking, and teasing in class). Parents can also influence the school to be more motivating.

MINIMIZE FRUSTRATIONS

The language-disordered child needs help in feeling important and avoiding frustrations. He needs to feel he will be listened to when he expresses his feelings. A positive attitude is necessary, and teasing and sarcasm are to be avoided. While success is good, the language-disordered child needs to feel good about himself even if he is not succeeding.

Parents can help the child avoid frustrations by encouraging controlled release of energy in nonharmful ways (e.g., planned exercise or household tasks requiring energy). The older child can be encouraged to retreat to his room to cool off and compose himself. Parents should avoid nagging and should positively reinforce purposeful activity. With older children, written "contracts" can be helpful to encourage behaviors without nagging.

Psychiatric Intervention

Children with developmental speech and language disorders are at risk for psychiatric disorders. However, it should be stressed that no particular psychiatric disorder is "characteristic" of these children. As in the case of children without developmental speech and language disorders, treatment planning in child psychiatry requires a detailed, comprehensive psychiatric evaluation.

Treatment Planning

Since treatment planning is dependent upon diagnosis, a comprehensive psychiatric evaluation is always required (Cantwell, 1980). This diagnostic evaluation must consider a number of questions: Does the child have a significant problem in development, manifested as an abnormality in behavior, emotions, relationships, or cognition, that is of sufficient severity and/or duration to cause distress, disability, or disadvantage? Does the clinical picture of the child's disorder fit a known and recognized clinical syndrome? Since most psychiatric disorders in childhood are of multifactorial etiology, what are the relative effects of familial, social, and biological factors in this child? What forces are currently maintaining the child's problem? What forces facilitate the child's normal development? What are the child's and the family's strengths and competencies? What is the probable untreated outcome of this disorder (considering the natural history of the clinical syndrome and also the data particular to the patient)? Is intervention necessary? What types of intervention are most likely to be effective?

The natural history of the disorder determines how urgent intervention is. It is much more important to intervene in a disorder that, untreated, is likely to have a disabling outcome than in a disorder that, untreated, will leave few residual effects. For a treatment to be considered efficacious, the outcome should be better than could be predicted from the untreated natural history.

Child psychiatry has no unifying underlying theoretical

orientation that is subscribed to by all practitioners, but, rather, is characterized by a wide variety of theoretical orientations. Therefore, it is not surprising that there are a variety of treatment approaches. Our conceptualization is that psychiatric disorders in childhood, with rare exceptions, are of multifactorial etiology, with contributions from interpersonal, biological, social, and other forces, and that multimodal treatment interventions may accordingly be most effective.

Treatment Illustration: Attention Deficit Disorder

A complete discussion of therapeutic intervention is beyond the scope of this chapter and can be found elsewhere (Cantwell, 1984). Here we illustrate treatment of the psychiatric disorder occurring most frequently in children with developmental speech and language disorders—namely, attention deficit disorder. The intervention principles outlined here are applicable to all children with developmental speech and language disorders, although treatment focus may differ from child to child. The essential feature of attention deficit disorder with hyperactivity is a chronic pattern of major difficulties with motor activity, impulsivity, and inattention, beginning early in life.

FAMILY INVOLVEMENT

It is our feeling that successful treatment begins with involvement of the family. Parents should be taught the nature and phenomenology of the syndrome, together with principles for structuring the child's environment and limiting his behavior. Much can be accomplished with simple environmental manipulation. The importance of avoiding overstimulation, excessive fatigue, and situations known to cause difficulty should be emphasized.

There are certain reading materials that are valuable for parents of children with attention deficit disorder. We recommend Wender and Wender (1978) and Stewart and Olds (1973). Referral of the family to organizations such as the local chapter of the National Association of Children with Learning

Disabilities may be useful; such organizations provide information on community resources, as well as group support. Programmed texts written for parents (Patterson, 1971; Patterson & Gullion, 1971) describe the basics of behavior intervention. The more extensive effort and professional involvement of larger "formal" behavior modification programs are not always required.

Studies of parents of children who have attention deficit disorder with hyperactivity suggest that a number of these parents may themselves have psychopathology in the attention deficit or "antisocial spectrum" areas; treatment for them may be necessary also. Children with this syndrome call forth the worst types of behavior from any parent; more formal family therapy may be required.

MEDICATIONS

Next, the use of stimulant medications or tricyclic antidepressants such as imipramine should be considered. Barkley's (1977) review suggests that about three-quarters of all children who have attention deficit disorder with hyperactivity show a positive response to one of the central nervous system stimulants (methylphenidate, magnesium pemoline, or one of the amphetamines). A similar percentage of cases in controlled studies have been found to respond positively to tricyclic antidepressants. However, these medications are clearly second choice to stimulants, since they are potentially more toxic and may be less successful for long-term usage due to development of tolerance over time.

There are limited data available regarding the "best" choice among the three major groups of stimulants. Children may have more side effects with, or may respond less well to, one stimulant than another. Thus, it is worthwhile to switch medications to determine which is most beneficial. There are earlier favorable reports suggesting that deanol and caffeine are effective with this syndrome; however, these reports have not been replicated in systematic controlled studies.

The stimulants, like all medications, affect many functions, including cognition, activity level, behavior, and academic achievement. Evidence suggests that the stimulants positively affect such cognitive functions as attention, perception, and memory; may influence cognitive style; and improve laboratory measures of learning.

In children with this syndrome who are positive responders to stimulants, the drugs have been found to produce a significant reduction in errors of omission during sustained performance tasks, as well as an increase in accuracy and vigilance on perceptual judgment tasks. These medications lead to more deliberate responses in reaction time tests, but they may also reduce latency and thus decrease reaction time. Stimulants also seem to affect the quality and quantity of motor activity. Thus, in a classroom setting, non-goal-directed motor activity will probably decrease, whereas in situations (such as the playground) where high levels of activity are appropriate, the activity level may remain constant or increase. The most consistent positive effect of stimulant medication is the reduction of disruptive and socially inappropriate behaviors.

Although earlier works found little evidence that stimulants positively affect problem-solving ability, classroom learning, or reasoning, more recent meta-analysis of the published data suggests otherwise. Current studies by Pelham and colleagues (1984) and Douglas and colleagues (1986) indicate that children who have attention deficit disorder with hyperactivity and developmental reading disorder, and receive stimulant medication, may demonstrate improved academic performance. Careful monitoring of positive and negative side effects, and assessment of the need for continuing treatment with medication, must be carried out on a regular basis.

The effects of the tricyclic antidepressants are similar to those of the stimulants with these children, although there are few data supporting the positive effect on cognitive functioning. Other medications are not likely to be effective for this disorder (Cantwell & Carlson, 1978).

BEHAVIOR MODIFICATION

Next, a formal behavior modification program should be considered for home and school. Behavior modification programs have been shown to be useful treatment adjuncts in reducing inappropriate behavior, increasing on-task behavior, and improving attention span (Gittelman-Klein *et al.*, 1976). It is important that expectations and reinforcements between home and school be consistent, and that attempts be made to generalize the behavioral program to academic tasks. Generalization should be built into the behavioral program so that techniques learned with one specific behavior can be applied to other behaviors that may arise.

Although the choice of behavior modification or medication is often described in the literature as an "either–or" decision, these treatment procedures should be considered as complementary. Successful behavior modification programs require involved parents and teachers who are willing to maintain consistency over time.

PSYCHOTHERAPY

The next issue is consideration of psychotherapy for the child and/or his family. As with other psychiatric disorders of childhood (Levitt, 1957, 1963; Rachman, 1971), evidence of the efficacy of individual psychotherapy for the core symptoms in attention deficit disorder is lacking. However, psychotherapy using active techniques such as those developed by R. Gardner (1973) may be indicated for secondary emotional symptoms, such as demoralization, depression, low self-esteem, or poor peer relationships. At the very least, the clinician should help the child to understand the nature of his difficulties and the ways in which other therapeutic interventions are intended to help the child help himself. In cases where the child with attention deficit disorder has become a "scapegoat" in a system of disturbed family interaction, a more dynamically oriented family approach may also be necessary. Studies (J. Satterfield, personal communication, 1984) have shown that a multimodality treatment program involving a combination of stimulant medication, behavior modification at the home and school, individual educational therapy, group therapy for the parents and child, and individual therapy for the child produces major changes in behavior and academic achievement over a 3-year period of time.

Attention deficit disorder with hyperactivity, like other conditions with no known etiology, has had a variety of different therapeutic techniques proposed for it. Most of these techniques have little scientific support. For example, interventions such as diets and vitamin combinations have received great media attention, even though there is little scientific evidence of their effectiveness. However, it is important for the clinician to be aware of the latest "therapeutic fads," since it is likely that families will have heard about them and will be seeking guidelines as to which of these are effective or ineffective.

SPECIFIC TREATMENT MODIFICATIONS

The discussion above considers the in-general treatment of children who have attention deficit disorder with hyperactivity. Obviously, treatment plans may have to be modified when applied to a child who also has developmental speech and language disorders. The speech and language disorders may interfere with the child's ability to participate in a psychotherapeutic program; in addition, a behavior modification program may have to be spelled out in more simplified fashion with such a child. There are no systematic studies of the effect of medication on attention deficit disorder with hyperactivity in children with developmental speech and language disorders; while there is no reason necessarily to believe that the response rate will be any different in these children, this is still possible. Based on the available evidence, a medication trial is as valid in these children as in children without developmental speech and language disorders, provided they meet the syndrome's core criteria of symptom pattern, age of onset, and chronicity.

Our studies and those of others suggest that in addition to attention deficit disorder with hyperactivity, other overt behavior disorders, such as oppositional disorder and conduct disorder, may be relatively common in children with developmental speech and language disorders. In addition, a substantial minority of these children (20% or so in our study) may have one or more of the anxiety disorders, such as generalized anxiety disorder or separation anxiety disorder. Different therapeutic modalities discussed in detail elsewhere (Cantwell, 1984) are necessary for these anxious children. Finally, to our knowledge, no study has ever examined various types of interventions (psychiatric intervention alone, speech and language intervention alone, or a combination of psychiatric and language interventions) with groups of children matched for psychiatric and linguistic diagnoses. This is an area for future research.

REFERENCES

Achenbach, T. (1978). The Child Behavior Profile. *Journal of Consulting and Clinical Psychology, 46*, 478–488.

Achenbach, T. (1985). *Youth self report.* Unpublished manuscript, University of Vermont, Department of Psychiatry.

Adler, S. (1964). *The nonverbal child.* Springfield, IL: Charles C. Thomas.

Alajouanine, T., & Lhermitte, F. (1965). Acquired aphasia in children. *Brain, 88*, 653–662.

Albright, R. W., & Albright, J. B. (1956). The phonology of a two-year-old child. *Word, 12*, 382–390.

American Association on Mental Deficiency. (1983). *Manual on terminology and classification.* Willimantic, CT: Author.

American Psychiatric Association. (1980). *Diagnostic and statistical manual of mental disorders* (3rd ed.). Washington, DC: Author.

Ammons, R., & Ammons, H. (1958). *Full Range Picture Vocabulary Test.* Missoula, MT: Psychological Test Specialists.

Ando, H., & Yoshimura, J. (1978). Prevalence of maladaptive behavior in retarded children as a function of IQ and age. *Journal of Abnormal Child Psychology, 6*, 345–349.

Andreasen, N. C. (1979). Thought, language, and communication disorders: 1. Clinical assessment, definition of terms and evaluation of their reliability. *Archives of General Psychiatry, 36*, 1325–1330.

Andreasen, N. C. (1982). There may be a schizophrenic language. *Behavioral and Brain Sciences, 5*, 588–589.

Anglin, J. (1970). *The growth of word meanings.* Cambridge, MA: M.I.T. Press.

Annett, M. (1981). The right-shift theory of handedness and developmental language problems. *Bulletin of the Orton Society, 31*, 103–121.

Aram, D. M., Ekelman, B., & Nation, J. E. (1984). Preschoolers with language disorders: 10 years later. *Journal of Speech and Hearing Research, 27*, 232–244.

Aram, D. M., & Nation, J. E. (1975). Patterns of language behavior in children with developmental language disorder. *Journal of Speech and Hearing Research, 18*, 229–241.

Aram, D. M., & Nation, J. E. (1980). Preschool language disorders and subsequent language and academic difficulties. *Journal of Communication Disorders, 13*, 159–170.

Aram, D. M., & Nation, J. E. (1982). *Child language disorders.* St. Louis: C. V. Mosby.

Baker, H. J., & Leland, B. (1967). *Detroit Tests of Learning Aptitude (DTLA).* Indianapolis, IN: Bobbs-Merrill.

Baker, L., & Cantwell, D. P. (1982). Psychiatric disorder in children with different types of communication disorders. *Journal of Communication Disorders, 15*, 113–126.

Baker, L., & Cantwell, D. P. (1984a). Developmental arithmetic disorder. In H. Kapland & B. Sadock (Eds.), *Comprehensive textbook of psychiatry IV* (pp. 1697–1699). Baltimore: Williams & Wilkins.

Baker, L., & Cantwell, D. P. (1984b). Developmental, social, and behavioral characteristics of speech and language disordered children. In S. Chess & A. Thomas (Eds.), *Annual Progress in Child Psychiatry & Child Development 1983* (pp. 205–216). New York: Brunner/Mazel.

Baker, L., & Cantwell, D. P. (1985). Psychiatric and learning disorders in children with speech and language disorders: A critical review. *Advances in Learning and Behavioral Disabilities, 4*, 1–28.

Baker, L., & Cantwell, D. P. (in press-a). Comparison of well, emotionally disordered, and behaviorally disordered children with linguistic problems. *Journal of the American Academy of Child Psychiatry.*

Baker, L., & Cantwell, D. P. (in press-b). Factors associated with psychiatric illness in at risk children. *Journal of Autism.*

Baker, L., & Cantwell, D. P., Rutter, M., & Bartak, L. (1976). Language and autism. In E. Ritvo (Ed.), *Autism: Diagnosis, current research, and management* (pp. 121–149). New York: Spectrum.

Baltaxe, C., & Simmons, J. Q. (1975). Language in childhood psychosis: A review. *Journal of Speech and Hearing Disorders, 40*, 439–458.

Bandler, R., & Grinder, J. (1979). *Frogs into princes: neurolinguistic programming.* Moab, UT: Real People Press.

Bangs, J. (1942). A clinical analysis of articulatory defects of the feeble minded. *Journal of Speech and Hearing Disorders, 7*, 343–356.

Bangs, T. E. (1975). *Vocabulary Comprehension Scale.* Boston: Teaching Resources.

Bankson, N. W. (1977). *Bankson Language Screening Test.* Baltimore: University Park Press.

Barkley, R. (1977). A review of stimulant drug research with hyperactive children. *Journal of Child Psychology and Psychiatry and Allied Disciplines, 18*, 137–165.

Barkley, R. (1981). Learning disabilities. In E. Mash & L. Terdal (Eds.), *Behavioral assessment of childhood disorders* (pp. 441–482). New York: Guilford Press.

Barrie-Blackley, S. (1973). Six-year-old children's understanding of sentences conjoined with time adverbs. *Journal of Psycholinguistic Research, 2*, 153–165.

Bartak, L., Rutter, M., & Cox, A. (1975). Comparative study of infantile autism and specific developmental receptive language disorder: I. The children. *British Journal of Psychiatry, 7*, 127–145.

Bartak, L., Rutter, M., Cox, A., & Newman, S. (1972). *Comparison of autism and aphasia.* Paper presented to the Social Sciences Research Council, London, England.

Bartolucci, G., & Albers, R. (1974). Deictic categories in the language of autistic children. *Journal of Autism and Childhood Schizophrenia, 14*, 131–141.

Bateson, M. C. (1975). Mother–infant exchanges: The epigenesis of conversational interaction. *Annals of the New York Academy of Sciences, 263*, 101–113.

Bax, M., Hart, H., & Jenkins, S. (1980). Assessment of speech and language development in the young child. *Pediatrics, 66*, 350–354.

Becker, W. (1971). *Parents are teachers.* Champaign, IL: Research Press.

Beitchman, J. (1983). Childhood schizophrenia: A review and comparison with adult onset schizophrenia. *Psychiatric Journal of the University of Ottawa, 8*(2), 25–37.

Beitchman, J. (1985). *Children's Self-Rating Scale.* Unpublished manuscript, Park Institute, Division of Child Psychiatry, Toronto.

Bellamy, M. M., & Bellamy, S. E. (1970). The acquisition of morphological inflections by children four to ten. *Language Learning, 20*, 199–121.

Blank, M., Rose, S. A., & Berlin, L. J. (1978). *Preschool Language Assessment Instrument: The language of learning in practice.* New York: Grune & Stratton.

Bleuler, E. (1950). *Dementia praecox or the group of schizophrenias* (J. Zinkin, Trans.). New York: International Universities Press.

Bliss, L., Allen, D., & Walker, G. (1978). Sentence structure of trainable and educable mentally retarded subjects. *Journal of Speech and Hearing Research, 21*, 722–731.

Bloodstein, O. (1979). *Speech pathology: An introduction*. Boston: Houghton Mifflin.

Bloom, L. (1970). *Language development: Form and function in emerging grammars*. Cambridge, MA: M.I.T. Press.

Bloom, L. (1973). Why not pivot grammar? In C. A. Ferguson & D. J. Slobin (Eds.), *Studies of child language development* (pp. 430–440). New York: Holt, Rinehart & Winston.

Bloom, L. (1978). The integration of form, content, and use in language development. In J. Kavanagh & W. Strange (Eds.), *Speech and language in the laboratory, school, and clinic* (pp. 210–246). Cambridge, MA: M.I.T. Press.

Bloom, L., & Lahey, M. (1978). *Language development and language disorders*. New York: Wiley.

Bloom, L., Rocissano, L., & Hood, L. (1976). Adult-child discourse: Developmental interaction between information processing and linguistic knowledge. *Cognitive Psychology, 8*, 521–552.

Boder, E. (1973). Developmental dyslexia: A diagnostic approach based on three atypical reading and spelling patterns. *Developmental Medicine and Childhood Neurology, 15*, 663–687.

Boehm, A. (1971). *Boehm Test of Basic Concepts*. New York: Psychological Corporation.

Bonvillian, J. D., Charrow, V. R., & Nelson, K. E. (1973). Psycholinguistic and educational implications of deafness. *Human Development, 16*, 321–345.

Bonvillian, J., Nelson, K., & Charrow, V. (1978). Languages and language related skills in deaf and hearing children. *Sign Language Studies, 12*, 211–250.

Boucher, J. (1976). Is autism primarily a language disorder? *British Journal of Disorders of Communication, 11*(2), 135–143.

Boucher, J. (1981). Memory for recent events in autistic children. *Journal of Autism and Developmental Disorders, 11*, 293–301.

Bowerman, M. (1978). Words and sentences: Uniformity, individual variation, and shifts over time in patterns of acquisition. In F. D. Minifie & L. L. Lloyd (Eds.), *Communicative and cognitive abilities: Early behavioral assessment* (pp. 349–396). Baltimore: University Park Press.

Braine, M. D. S. (1963). The ontogeny of English phrase structure: The first phrase. *Language, 39*, 1–13.

Brandes, P., & Ehinger, D. (1981). The effects of early middle ear pathology on auditory perception and academic achievement. *Journal of Speech and Hearing Disorders, 46*, 301–307.

Brannon, J., Jr. (1968). A comparison of syntactic structures in the speech of three and four year old children. *Language and Speech, 11*, 171–181.

Brenza, B., Kricos, P., & Lasky, E. (1981). Comprehension and production of basic semantic concepts of older hearing-impaired children. *Journal of Speech and Hearing Research, 40*, 414–419.

Brimer, M. A., & Dunn, L. M. (1962). *English Picture Vocabulary Test*. Bristol, England: Educational Evaluation Enterprises.

Brown, B. B. (1973). Language disorders in children. *Public Health, 87*(4), 115–118.

Brown, R. (1978). The original word game. In L. Bloom (Ed.), *Readings in language development* (pp. 384–389). New York: Wiley.

Bryan, T., Donahue, M., & Pearl, R. (1981). Learning disabled children's peer interactions during a small group problem solving task. *Learning Disabilities Quarterly, 4*, 13–22.

Bryen, D., & Gerber, A. (1981). Assessing language and its use. In D. Bryen &

A. Gerber (Eds.), *Language and Learning Disabilities* (pp. 115–158). Baltimore: Williams & Wilkins.

Bryson, C. (1970). Systematic identification of perceptual disabilities in autistic children. *Perceptual and Motor Skills, 31*, 239–246.

Bryson, C. (1972). Short term memory and cross modal information processing in autistic children. *Journal of Learning Disabilities, 5*, 81–91.

Bzoch, K. R., & League, R. L. (1970). *Receptive–Expressive–Emergent Language Scale for the measurement of language skills in infancy*. Baltimore: University Park Press.

Campbell, T., & Heaton, E. (1978). An expressive speech program for a child with acquired aphasia: A case study. *Canadian Journal of Human Communication, Summer*, 89–102.

Cantwell, D. P. (1980). The diagnostic process and diagnostic classification in child psychiatry—DSM-III. *Journal of the American Academy of Child Psychiatry, 19*, 345–355.

Cantwell, D. P. (1984). Psychiatric disorders. In S. Gellis & B. Kagan (Eds.), *Current pediatric therapy* (pp. 14–19). Philadelphia: W. B. Saunders.

Cantwell, D. P., & Baker, L. (1977). Psychiatric disorder in children with speech and language retardation: A critical review. *Archives of General Psychiatry, 34*, 583–591.

Cantwell, D. P., & Baker, L. (1980a). Academic failures in children with communication disorders. *Journal of the American Academy of Child Psychiatry, 19*, 579–591.

Cantwell, D. P., & Baker, L. (1980b). Psychiatric and behavioral characteristics of children with communication disorders. *Journal of Pediatric Psychology, 5*, 161–178.

Cantwell, D. P., & Baker, L. (1983). Depression in children with speech, language, and learning disorders. *Journal of Children in Contemporary Society, 15*, 51–59.

Cantwell, D. P., & Baker, L. (1985). Psychiatric and learning disorders in children with speech and language disorders: A descriptive analysis. *Advances in Learning and Behavioral Disabilities, 4*, 29–47.

Cantwell, D. P., & Baker, L. (in press). Prevalence and type of psychiatric disorder and developmental disorder in three speech and language groups. *Journal of Communication Disorders*.

Cantwell, D. P., Baker, L., & Rutter, M. (1978). A comparative study of infantile autism and specific developmental receptive language disorder. IV. An analysis of syntax and language functioning. *Journal of Child Psychology and Psychiatry and Allied Disciplines, 19*, 351–362.

Cantwell, D. P., & Carlson, G. (1978). Stimulants. In J. Werry (Ed.), *Pediatric psychopharmacology—the use of behavior modifying drugs in children* (pp. 171–207). New York: Brunner/Mazel.

Capute, A. J., & Accardo, P. J. (1978). Linguistic and auditory milestones during the first two years of life. *Clinical Pediatrics, 17*(11), 847–852.

Carrow, E. (1972). Assessment of speech and language in children. In J. E. McLean, D. E. Yoder, & R. L. Schiefelbusch (Eds.), *Language intervention with the retarded: Developing strategies* (pp. 52–88). Baltimore: University Park Press.

Carrow, E. (1974a). *Austin Spanish Articulation Test (ASAT)*. Boston: Teaching Resources Corporation.

Carrow, E. (1974b). *Carrow Elicited Language Inventory*. New York: Teaching Resources.

Carrow, E. (1978). *Test of Auditory Comprehension of Language (TACL)*. Austin, TX: Learning Concepts.

Carrow-Woodfolk, E., & Lynch, J. (1982). *An integrative approach to language disorders in chidren*. New York: Grune & Stratton.

Cazden, C. (1965). *Environmental assistance to the child's acquisition of grammar*. Unpublished doctoral dissertation, Harvard Graduate School of Education.

Chapanis, L. (1977). Language deficits and cross modal sensory perception. In S. Segalowitz & F. Gruber (Eds.), *Language development and neurological theory* (pp. 107–120). New York: Academic Press.

Chapman, D., & Nation, J. (1981). Patterns of language performance in educable mentally retarded children. *Journal of Communication Disorders, 14*, 245–254.

Chapman, R. (1978). Comprehension strategies in children. In J. F. Kavanagh & W. Strange (Eds.), *Speech and language in the laboratory, school, and clinic* (pp. 308–327). Cambridge, MA: M.I.T. Press.

Chapman, R., & Miller, J. F. (1975). Word order in early two and three word utterances: Does production precede comprehension? *Journal of Speech and Hearing Research, 18*, 355–371.

Chappell, G. E. (1970). Developmental aphasia revisited. *Journal of Communication Disorders, 3*, 181–197.

Chase, R. (1972). Neurological aspects of language disorders in children. In J. V. Irwin & M. Marge (Eds.), *Principles of childhood language disabilities* (pp. 96–136). Englewood Cliffs, NJ: Prentice-Hall.

Chess, S., & Fernandez, P. (1980). Do deaf children have a typical personality? *Journal of the American Academy of Child Psychiatry, 19*, 654–664.

Chomsky, C. (1969). *The acquisition of language from five to ten.* Cambridge, MA: MIT Press.

Clark, H. H. (1977). Inferences in comprehension. In D. L. LaBerge & S. J. Samuels (Eds.), *Basic processes in reading: Perception and comprehension* (pp. 243–264). Hillsdale, NJ: Erlbaum.

Clark, H. H., & Clark, E. V. (1977). *Psychology and language: An introduction to linguistics.* New York: Harcourt Brace Jovanovich.

Clements, J., Evans, C., Jones, C., Osborne, K., & Upton, G. (1982). Evaluation of a home-based language training programme with severely mentally handicapped children. *Behaviour Research and Therapy, 20*, 243–249.

Cohen, D., Caparulo, B., & Shaywitz, B. (1976). Primary childhood aphasia and childhood autism: Clinical, biological and conceptual observations. *Journal of the American Academy of Child Psychiatry, 4*, 604–645.

Condon, W. (1975). Multiple responses to sound in dysfunctional children. *Journal of Autism and Childhood Schizophrenia, 5*, 37–56.

Conners, C. K., & Barkley, R. A. (1985). Rating scales and checklists for child psychopharmacology. *Psychopharmacology Bulletin, 21*, 809–815.

Cooper, J., & Ferry, P. (1978). Acquired auditory verbal agnosia of seizures in childhood. *Journal of Speech and Hearing Disorders, 43*, 176–184.

Cooper, J., & Griffiths, P. (1978). Treatment and prognosis. In M. Wyke (Ed.), *Developmental dysphasia* (pp. 159–176). New York: Academic Press.

Cooper, J., Moodley, M., & Reynell, J. (1979). The developmental language programme results from a five year study. *British Journal of Disorders of Communication, 14*, 57–69.

Costello, M. R. (1977). Evaluation of auditory behavior using the Flowers–Costello test for central auditory abilities. In R. W. Keith (Ed.), *Central auditory dysfunction* (pp. 257–276). New York: Grune & Stratton.

Cowan, P., Hoddinott, B., & Wright, B. (1965). Compliance and resistance in the conditioning of autistic children: An exploratory study. *Child Development, 36*, 913–923.

Crabtree, M. (1963). *The Houston Test for Language Development.* Houston, TX: Houston Test.

Crager, R. L. (1972). *Test of Concept Utilization (TCU).* Los Angeles: Western Psychological Services.

Cromer, R. F. (1980). Normal language development: Recent progress. In L. A. Hersov, M. Berger, & E. A. R. Nicol (Eds.), *Language and language disorders in childhood* (pp. 1-21). New York: Pergamon Press.

Crookes, T., & Greene, M. (1963). Some characteristics of children with two types of speech disorder. *British Journal of Educational Psychology, 33,* 31–40.

Cross, T. (1978). Mother's speech and its association with rate of linguistic development in young children. In C. Snow & W. Waterson (Eds.), *The development of communication* (pp. 119-216). New York: Wiley.

Culbertson, J. L., Norlin, P. F., & Ferry, P. C. (1981). Communication disorders in childhood. *Journal of Pediatric Psychology, 6,* 69–84.

Cunningham, M. (1968). A comparison of the language of psychotic and nonpsychotic children who are mentally retarded. *Journal of Child Psychology and Psychiatry and Allied Disciplines, 9,* 229–244.

Dailey, J. T. (1977). *Language Facility Test.* Alexandria, VA: Allington Corporation.

Dale, P. S. (1976). *Language development, structure, and function* (2nd ed.). New York: Holt, Rinehart & Winston.

Darley, F. L., & Winitz, H. (1961). Age of first word: Review of the research. *Journal of Speech and Hearing Disorders, 26,* 271–290.

Davis, H., & Kranz, F. (1964). The international standard reference zero for pure tone audiometers and its relations to the evaluation of impairment of hearing. *Journal of Speech and Hearing Research, 7,* 7–16.

Davis, S., & Marcus, L. (1980). Involving parents in the treatment of severely communication disordered children. *Journal of Pediatric Psychology, 5,* 189–198.

Dawson, G., Warrenburg, S., & Fuller, P. (1982). Cerebral lateralization in individuals diagnosed as autistic in early childhood. *Brain and Language, 15,* 353–368.

deAjuriaguerra, J., Jaeggi, A., Guignard, F., Kocher, F., Maquard, M., Roth, S., & Schmid, E. (1976). The development and prognosis of dysphasia in children. In D. Morehead & A. Morehead (Eds.), *Normal and deficient child language* (pp. 345–385). Baltimore: University Park Press.

DeHirsch, K. (1967). Language disturbances. In A. Freedman & M. Kaplan (Eds.), *Comprehensive textbook of psychiatry* (pp. 1376–1380). Baltimore: Williams & Wilkins.

DeHirsch, K. (1975). Language deficits in children with developmental lags. *Psychoanalytic Study of the Child, 30,* 95–126.

DeLong, G. (1978). A neuropsychologic interpretation of infantile autism. In M. Rutter & E. Schopler (Eds.), *Autism: A reappraisal of concepts and treatment* (pp. 207–217). New York: Plenum.

DeMeyer, M., Alpern, G., Barton, S., DeMeyer, W., Churchill, D., Hingtgen, J., Bryson, C., Pontius, W., & Kimberlin, C. (1972). Imitation in autistic, early schizophrenic, and nonpsychotic subnormal children. *Journal of Autism and Childhood Schizophrenia, 2,* 264–287.

Deonna, T., Beaumanior, A., Gaillard, F., & Assal, G. (1977). Acquired aphasia in childhood with seizure disorder: A heterogeneous syndrome. *Neuropaediatrie, 8,* 263–273.

Deonna, T., Fletcher, P., & Voumard, C. (1982). Temporal regression during language acquisition: A linguistic analysis of a 2½ year old child with epileptic aphasia. *Developmental Medicine and Child Neurology, 24,* 156–163.

DePaulo, B., & Bonvillian, J. (1978). The effect on language development of the special characteristics of speech addressed to children. *Journal of Psycholinguistic Research, 7,* 189–211.

Deuel, R. (1983). Aphasia in childhood. In H. Myklebust (Ed.), *Progress in learning disabilities* (Vol. 5, pp. 29–43). New York: Grune & Stratton.

De Villiers, P. A., & De Villiers, J. G. (1973). A cross-sectional study of the acquisition in child speech. *Journal of Psycholinguistic Research, 2,* 267–278.

De Villiers, J. G., & De Villiers, P. A. (1978). *Language Acquisition.* Cambridge: Harvard University Press.

DiSimoni, F. (1978). *The Token Test for Children.* Boston: Teaching Resources Corporation.

Donahue, M. L. (1981). Requesting strategies of learning disabled children. *Applied Psycholinguistics, 2,* 213–234.

Douglas, V. I., Barr, R. G., O'Neill, M. E., & Britton, B. G. (1986). Short-term effects of methylphenidate on the cognitive, learning, and academic performance of children with attention deficit disorder in the laboratory and the classroom. *Journal of Child Psychology & Psychiatry, 27,* 191–212.

Downs, M. (1977). The expanding imperatives of early identification. In F. Bess (Ed.), *Childhood deafness* (pp. 95–106). New York: Grune & Stratton.

Drumwright, A. F. (1971). *The Denver Articulation Screening Exam (DASE).* Denver: University of Colorado Medical Center.

Dunn, L. M., & Dunn, L. M. (1981). *Peabody Picture Vocabulary Test (PPVT).* (rev. ed.). Circle Pines, MN: American Guidance Services.

Eggers, C. (1978). Course and prognosis of childhood schizophrenia. *Journal of Autism and Childhood Schizophrenia, 8,* 21–36.

Eisenson, J. (1963). Disorders of language in children. *Journal of Pediatrics, 62,* 20–24.

Eisenson, J. (1966). Perceptual disturbances in children with central nervous system dysfunctions and implications for language development. *British Journal of Disorders of Communication, 1,* 21–32.

Eisenson, J. (1968). Developmental aphasia: A speculative view with therapeutic implications. *Journal of Speech and Hearing Disorders, 33,* 3–13.

Eisenson, J. (1972). *Aphasia in children.* New York: Harper & Row.

Eisenson, J., & Ingram, D. (1972). Childhood aphasia: An updated concept based on recent research. *Acta Symbolica, 3,* 108–116.

Eisenson, J., & Ogilvie, M. (1983). *Communicative disorders in children* (5th ed.). New York: Macmillan.

Elson, A., Pearson, C., Jones, C., & Schumaker, E. (1965). Follow-up study of childhood elective mutism. *Archives of General Psychiatry, 13,* 182–187.

Englemann, S. E. (1967). *The Basic Concept Inventory.* Chicago: Follett.

Ensminger, E., & Smith, J. (1965). Language development and the ITPA. *Training School Bulletin, 62,* 97–107.

Farmer, A., & Goldsworthy, C. (1982, March). *A neuropsychological model for treatment of language disorders, learning disabilities, and aphasia.* Paper presented at the meeting of the California State American Speech and Hearing Association, Monterey.

Fay, W. H. (1971). On normal and autistic pronouns. *Jounral of Speech and Hearing Disorders, 36,* 242–249.

Fay, W. H. (1980). The examinations of speech, language and hearing, part a. In P. LaBenz & E. LaBenz (Eds.), *Early correlates of speech, language, and hearing* (pp. 28–30). Littleton, MA: P.S.G.

Fay, W. H., & Anderson, D. (1981). Children's echo-reactions as a function of increasing lexical difficulty: A developmental study. *Journal of Genetic Psychology, 138,* 259–267.

Feighner, J., Robins, E., Guze, S., Woodruff, R., Winokur, G., & Muñoz, R. (1972). Diagnostic criteria for use in psychiatric research. *Archives of General Psychiatry, 26,* 57–63.

Fein, D., Skoff, B., & Mirsky, A. (1981). Clinical correlates of brain stem dysfunction in autistic children. *Journal of Autism and Developmental Disorders, 11,* 303–315.

Feldman, C., & Rodgon, M. (1970). *The effects of various types of adult response in the syntactic acquisition of 2 to 3 year olds.* Unpublished manuscript, University of Chicago, Psychology Department.

Ferguson, C. A. (1978). Learning to pronounce: The earliest stages of phonological development in the child. In F. D. Minifie & L. L. Lloyd (Eds.), *Communicative and cognitive abilities: Early behavioral assessment* (pp. 273–297). Baltimore: University Park Press.

Filer, P. (1981). Conversations with language delayed children: How to get them talking. *Academic Therapy, 17,* 57–63.

Fisher, H., & Logemann, J. 1971). *The Fisher–Logemann Test of Articulation Competence.* Boston: Houghton Mifflin.

Flowers, A. (1972). *Short term auditory retrieval and storage.* Dearborn, MI: Perceptual Learning Systems.

Flowers, A. (1975). *Flowers Auditory Test of Selective Attention* (experimental ed.). Dearborn, MI: Perceptual Learning Systems.

Flowers, A., Costello, M. R., & Small, V. (1970). *Flowers–Costello Test of Central Auditory Abilities.* Dearborn, MI: Perceptual Learning Systems.

Fontana, D., & Diaper, R. (1981). Effects of a special remedial movement program upon linguistic development in ESN boys. *Educational Psychology, 1,* 261–266.

Forness, S., & Kavale, K. (1983a). Remediation of reading disabilities: Part 1. Issues and concepts. *Learning Disabilities, 2,* 141–152.

Forness, S., & Kavale, K. (1983b). Remediation of reading disabilities: Part 2. Classification and approaches. *Learning Disabilities, 2,* 153–164.

Foster, R., Giddan, J. J., & Stark, J. (1973). *Assessment of Children's Language Comprehension (ACLC)* (rev. ed.). Palo Alto, CA: Counseling Psychologists Press.

Fraser, C., Bellugi, U., & Brown, R. (1963). Control of grammar: Imitation, comprehension, and production. *Journal of Verbal Learning and Verbal Behavior, 2,* 121–135.

Freeman, R. (1977). Psychiatric aspects of sensory disorders and intervention. In P. Graham (Ed.), *Epidemiological approaches in child psychiatry* (pp. 275–304). London: Academic Press.

Fristoe, M. (1976). Communication assessment in the mentally retarded. In P. Mittler (Ed.), *Research to practice in mental retardation* (Vol. 2, pp. 207–216). Baltimore: University Park Press.

Frith, U. (1969). Emphasis and meaning recall in normal and autistic children. *Language and Speech, 12,* 28–38.

Frumkin, B. A., & Rapin, I. (1979). *Perception of vowels and consonant–vowels of varying duration in language–impaired children.* Paper presented at the meeting of the International Neuropsychology Society, New York.

Fudala, J. B. (1974). *Arizona Articulation Proficiency Scale.* Los Angeles: Western Psychological Services.

Fudala, J. B., Kunze, L. H., & Ross, J. D. (1974). *Auditory Pointing Test.* San Rafael, CA: Academic Therapy.

Fulton, R., & Lloyd, L. (1968). Hearing impairment in a population of children with Down's syndrome. *American Journal of Mental Deficiency, 73,* 298–302.

Fundudis, T., Kolvin, I., & Garside, R. (1980). A follow-up of speech retarded children. In L. Hersov, M. Berger, & A. Nicol (Eds.), *Language and language disorders in childhood* (pp. 97–114). New York: Pergamon Press.

Furth, H. G. (1961). The influence of language on the development of concept formation in deaf children. In P. Adams (Ed.), *Language in thinking: Selected readings* (pp. 50–57). Baltimore: Penguin Books.

Furth, H. L. (1971). Linguistic deficiency and thinking research with deaf subjects 1964–1969. *Psychological Bulletin, 76,* 58–72.

Gall, F. (1825). *On the function of the brain and each of its parts* (Vols. 1–6). Boston: March, Capen & Lyon.

Gardner, H., Kircher, M., Winner, E., & Parkins, D. (1975). Children's metaphoric productions and preferences. *Journal of Child Language, 2*, 125–141.

Gardner, M. F. (1979). *Expressive One-Word Picture Vocabulary Test*. Novato, CA: Academic Therapy.

Gardner, R. (1973). Psychotherapy of the psychogenic problems secondary to minimal brain dysfunction. *International Journal of Child Psychotherapy, 2*, 224–256.

Garvey, C., & Berninger, G. (1981). Timing and turn taking in children's conversations. *Discourse Processes, 4*, 27–58.

Garvey, M., & Gordon, N. (1973). A follow-up study of children with disorders of speech development. *British Journal of Disorders of Communication, 8*, 17–28.

Gascon, C., Victor, D., Lombroso, C., & Goodglass, H. (1973). Language disorders, convulsive disorder and electroencephalographic abnormalities acquired syndrome in children. *Archives of Neurology, 28*, 156–162.

Geers, A., & Moog, J. (1978). Syntactic maturity of spontaneous speech and elicited imitations of hearing impaired children. *Journal of Speech and Hearing Disorders, 43*, 380–391.

Georgetown University Hospital, Division of communication disorders. (1978) *Speech and language screening*. Unpublished manuscript.

Gerard, J., & Weinstock, G. (1981). *Language Proficiency Test (LPT)*. Novato, CA: Academic Therapy.

German, D. (1979). Word finding skills in children with learning disabilities. *Journal of Learning Disabilities, 12*, 43–48.

Gittleman-Klein, R., Klein, D., Abikoff, H., Katz, S., Gloisten, A., & Kates, W. (1967). Relative efficacy of methylphenidate and behavior modification in hyperkinetic children: An interim report. *Journal of Abnormal Child Psychology, 4*, 361–379.

Goda, S. (1970). *Articulation therapy and consonant drill book*. New York: Grune & Stratton.

Goldberg, B., Lobb, H., & Krou, H. (1975). Psychiatric problems of the deaf child. *Canadian Psychiatric Association Journal, 20*, 75–83.

Goldman, R., & Fristoe, M. (1972). *Goldman–Fristoe Test of Articulation (GFTA)*. (rev. ed.). Circle Pines, MN: American Guidance Service.

Goldman, R., Fristoe, M., & Woodcock, R. (1970). *Goldman–Fristoe–Woodcock Test of Auditory Discrimination*. Circle Pines, MN: American Guidance Service.

Goldman, R., Fristoe, M., & Woodcock, R. (1974). *Goldman–Fristoe–Woodcock Sound Symbol Test*. Circle Pines, MN: American Guidance Service.

Goldman, R., Fristoe, M., & Woodcock, R. (1976). *Goldman–Fristoe–Woodcock Auditory Selective Attention Test*. Circle Pines, MN: American Guidance Service.

Goldstein, M. N. (1974). Auditory agnosia for speech (pure word deafness). *Brain and Language, 1*, 195–204.

Golinkoff, R. M. (Ed.). (1983). *The transition from prelinguistic to linguistic communication*. Hillsdale, NJ: Erlbaum.

Gordan, W. L., & Panagos, J. M. (1976). Developmental transformation capacity of children with Down's syndrome. *Perceptual and Motor Skills, 43*, 967–973.

Gordon, N. (1966). The child who does not talk: Problems of diagnosis with special reference to children with severe auditory agnosia. *British Journal of Disorders of Communication, 1*, 78–84.

Graham, J., & Graham, L. (1971). Language behavior of the mentally retarded: Syntactic characteristics. *American Journal of Mental Deficiency, 75*, 623–629.

Gray, W. S. (1967). *Gray Oral Reading Tests*. Los Angeles: Western Psychological Services.

Greenfield, P., & Smith, J. (1976). *The structure of communication in early language development*. New York: Academic Press.

Griffiths, C. P. S. (1969). A follow-up study of children with disorders of speech. *British Journal of Disorders of Communication, 4*, 46–56.

Griffiths, P. (1972). *Developmental aphasia: An introduction*. London: Invalid Children's Aid Association.

Gualtieri, C., Adams, A., Shen, C., & Loiselle, D. (1982). Minor physical anomalies in alcoholic and schizophrenic adults and hyperactive and autistic children. *American Journal of Psychiatry, 139*, 640–643.

Guttman, E. (1942). Aphasia in children. *Brain, 65*, 205–219.

Hagen, C. (1981). Language disorders secondary to closed head injury: Diagnosis and treatment. *Topics in Language Disorders, 1*(4), 13–87.

Hall, P., & Tomblin, J. (1978). A follow-up study of children with articulation and language disorders. *Journal of Speech and Hearing Disorders, 43*, 227–241.

Hammill, D. D., & Larsen, S. C. (1974). The effectiveness of psycholinguistic training. *Exceptional Children, 40*, 5–13.

Hammill, D. D., Brown, V. L., Larsen, S. C., & Wiederholt, J. L. (1980). *Test of Adolescent Language (TOAL): A multidimensional approach to assessment*. Austin, TX: Pro-Ed.

Hanson, D., & Gottesman, I. (1976). The genetics, if any, of infantile autism and childhood schizophrenia. *Journal of Autism and Childhood Schizophrenia, 6*, 209–234.

Hassibi, M., & Breuer, H. (1980). *Disordered thinking and communication*. New York: Plenum Press.

Hauser, S., DeLong, G., & Rosman, W. (1975). Pneumographic findings in the infantile autism syndrome. *Brain, 98*, 667–688.

Hecaen, H. (1976). Acquired aphasia in children and the ontogenesis of hemispheric functional specialization. *Brain and Language, 3*, 114–134.

Hedrick, D. L., Prather, E. M., & Tobin, A. R. (1975). *Sequenced Inventory of Communication Development*. Seattle: University of Washington Press.

Hejna, R. F. (1968). *Developmental Articulation Test*. Ann Arbor, MI: Speech Materials.

Hermelin, B. (1971). Rules and language. In M. Rutter (Ed.), *Infantile autism: Concepts, characteristics, and treatment* (pp. 98–112). London: Whitefriars Press.

Hetzler, B., & Griffin, J. (1981). Infantile autism and the temporal lobe of the brain. *Journal of Autism and Developmental Disorders, 11*, 317–330.

Hier, D., Lemay, M., & Rosenberger, P. (1979). Autism and unfavorable left–right asymmetries of the brain. *Journal of Autism and Developmental Disorders, 9*, 153–159.

Hingtgen, J., & Bryson, C. (1972). Recent developments in the study of early childhood psychosis: Infantile autism, childhood schizophrenia and related disorders. *Schizophrenia Bulletin, 5*, 8–55.

Hirshoren, A., & Schnittjer, C. (1979). Dimensions of problem behavior in deaf children. *Journal of Abnormal Child Psychology, 7*, 221–228.

Hiskey, M. S. (1966). *Hiskey–Nebraska Test of Learning Aptitude*. Lincoln, NE: Union College Press.

Hixson, P. H. (1979). Guidelines for recognizing delayed language development. *Ear, Nose, and Throat Journal, 58*(7), 310–315.

Hodson, B., & Paden, E. (1981). Phonological processes which characterize unintelligible and intelligible speech in early childhood. *Journal of Speech and Hearing Disorders, 46*, 369–373.

Homzie, M. J., & Lindsay, J. S. (1984). Language and the young stutterer. *Brain and Language, 22*, 232–252.

Howells, J., & Guirguis, W. (1984). Childhood schizophrenia twenty years later. *Archives of General Psychiatry, 41*, 123–128.

Howie, V., Ploussard, J., & Sloyer, J. (1976). Natural history of otitis media. *Annals of Otology, Rhinology, and Laryngology, 25*(18), 2–8.

Howlin, P. (1980). Language. In M. Rutter (Ed.), *Scientific foundations of developmental psychiatry* (pp. 198–219). London: Heinemann.

Hresko, W. P., Reid, D. K., & Hammill, D. D. (1981). *Test of Early Language Development (TELD)*. Austin, TX: Pro-Ed.

Hubbell, R. (1977). On facilitating spontaneous talking in young children. *Journal of Speech and Hearing Disorders, 42*, 216–231.

Humphrey, I., III, Knipstein, R., & Bumpass, E. (1975). Gradually developing aphasia in children: A diagnostic problem. *Journal of the American Academy of Child Psychiatry, 14*, 652–665.

Hursh, D., & Sherman, J. (1973). The effects of parent-presented models and praise on the vocal behavior of their children. *Journal of Exceptional Child Psychology, 15* 328–339.

Hurtig, R., Ensnid, S., & Toblin, J. (1982). The communicative function of question production in autistic children. *Journal of Autism and Developmental Disorders, 12*, 51–69.

Huttenlocher, P., & Huttenlocher, J. (1973). A study of children with hyperlexia. *Neuropsychologia, 23*, 1107–1116.

Ingram, D. (1972). *Phonological analysis of a developmentally aphasic child.* Unpublished manuscript, Scottish Rite Institute for Childhood Aphasia, Stanford, CA.

Ingram, D. (1976). *Phonological disability in children.* New York: Elsevier.

Jakobson, R. (1968). *Child language: Aphasia and phonological universals.* The Hague: Mouton.

Jastak, J. F., Bijou, S. W., & Jastak, S. R. (1976). *Wide Range Achievement Test.* Wilmington, DE: Guidance Assoc.

Johnson, D. (1981). Factors to consider in programming for children with language disorders. *Topics in Learning and Learning Disabilities, 1*(2), 13–27.

Johnston, J. R., & Kahmi, A. (1980). *The same can be less: Syntactic and semantic aspects of the utterances of language impaired children.* Paper presented at the First Annual Symposium on Research in Child Language Disorders, Madison, WI.

Johnston, J. R., & Schery, T. (1976). The use of grammatical morphemes by children with communicative disorders. In D. Morehead & A. Morehead (Eds.), *Normal and deficient child language* (pp. 239–258). Baltimore: University Park Press.

Jordan, L. (1980). Receptive and expressive language problems occurring in combination with a seizure disorder: A case report. *Journal of Communication Disorders, 13*, 295–303.

Jordan, T. (1967). Retrospective versus prospective techniques in research on learning disability. *Journal of Special Education, 13*, 257–265.

Kahn, L. (1982). A review of 16 major phonological processes. *Language, Speech, and Hearing Services in Schools, 13*(2), 77–85.

Kanner, L. (1946). Irrelevant and metaphorical language in early infantile autism. *American Journal of Psychiatry, 103*, 242–246.

Kanner, L. (1971). Follow-up study of 11 autistic children originally reported in 1943. *Journal of Autism and Childhood Schizophrenia, 1*, 119–145.

Kaplan, G. J., Fleshman, J. K., Bender, T. R., Baum, C., & Clark, P. S. (1973). Longterm effects of otitis media: A ten year cohort study of Alaskan Eskimo children. *Pediatrics, 52*, 577–585.

Karmiloff-Smith, A. (1979). *A functional approach to child language.* Cambridge, England: Cambridge University Press.

Kavale, K. (1981). Functions of the Illinois Test of Psycholinguistic Abilities (ITPA): Are they trainable? *Exceptional Children, 17*, 496–510.

Keane, V. (1972). The incidence of speech and language problems in the mentally retarded. *Mental Retardation, 10*(2), 3–8.

Keeley, S. M., Shemberg, K. M., & Carbonell, J. (1976). Operant clinical intervention: Behavior management or beyond? Where are the data? *Behavior Therapy, 7*, 292–303.

Keir, E. H. (1977). Auditory information processing and learning disabilities. In L. Tarnopol & M. Tarnopol (Eds.), *Brain function and reading disability* (pp. 147–176). Baltimore: University Park Press.

Keogh, K., Major-Kingsley, S., Omori-Gordon, H., & Reid, H. (1982). *A system of marker variables for the field of learning disabilities.* Syracuse, NY: Syracuse University Press.

Kimmell, E. M., & Wahl, J. (1969). *Screening Test for Auditory Perception.* San Rafael, CA: Academy Therapy.

King, R., Jones, C., & Lasky, E. (1982). In retrospect a 15 year follow-up of speech-language-disordered children. *Language, Speech, and Hearing Services in Schools, 13*, 24–32.

Kinsbourne, M. (1979). Language lateralization and developmental disorders. In C. L. Ludlow & M. E. Doran-Quine (Eds.), *The neurological bases of language disorders in children: Methods and directions for research* (pp. 91–108). Washington, DC: U.S. Department of Health, Education & Welfare.

Kinsbourne, M., & Caplan, P. (1979). *Children's learning and attentional problems.* Boston: Little, Brown.

Kirk, S. A., McCarthy, J. J., & Kirk, W. D. (1968). *The Illinois Test of Psycholinguistic Abilities (ITPA)* (rev. ed.). Urbana: University of Illinois Press.

Klackenberg, G. (1980). What happens to children with retarded speech at 3? Longitudinal study of a sample of normal infants up to twenty years of age. *Acta Paediatrica Scandinavica, 69*, 681–685.

Kolvin, I. (1971). Studies in childhood psychoses. *British Journal of Psychiatry, 118*, 381–419.

Kolvin, I., & Fundudis, T. (1981). Elective mute children: Psychological development and background factors. *Journal of Child Psychology, 22*, 219–232.

Koppitz, E. M. (1977). *The Visual Aural Digit Span Test (VADS).* New York: Grune & Stratton.

Kracke, I. (1975). Perception of rhythmic sequences by receptive aphasic and deaf children. *British Journal of Disorders of Communication, 10*, 43–51.

Kydd, R., & Werry, J. (1982). Schizophrenia in children under sixteen years. *Journal of Autism and Developmental Disorders, 12*, 343–357.

Lackner, J. (1968). Developmental study of language behavior in retarded children. *Neuropsychologia, 6*, 301–320.

Landau, W., Goldstein, R., & Kleffner, F. (1960). Congenital aphasia: A clinicopathologic study. *Neurology, 10*, 915–921.

Landau, W., Kleffner, F. (1957). Syndrome of acquired aphasia with convulsive disorder in children. *Neuropsychologia, 1*, 523–530.

Lasky, E. Z., & Tobin, H. (1973). Linguistic and non-linguistic competing message effects. *Journal of Learning Disabilities, 6*, 243–250.

Lee, L. (1966). Developmental sentence types: A method for comparing normal and deviant syntactic development. *Journal of Speech and Hearing Disorders, 31*, 311–330.

Lee, L. (1971). *Northwestern Syntax Screening Test (NSST).* Evanston, IL: Northwestern University Press.

Lee, L. (1974). *Developmental Sentence Analysis (DSA).* Evanston, IL: Northwestern University Press.

Lenneberg, E. (1967). *Biological foundations of language.* New York: Wiley.

Lenneberg, E., Nichols, I., & Rosenberger, E. (1964). Primitive stages of language development in mongolism. *Research Publications: Association for Research in Nervous and Mental Disease, 42*, 119–137.

Leonard, L. B. (1972). What is deviant language? *Journal of Speech and Hearing Disorders, 37*, 427–446.

Leonard, L. B. (1973). The nature of deviant articulation. *Journal of Speech and Hearing Disorders, 38*, 156–161.

Leonard, L. B., Schwartz, R. G., Folger, M. K., & Wilcox, M. J. (1978). Some aspects of child phonology in imitative and spontaneous speech. *Journal of Child Language, 5*, 403–415.

Lerea, L., & Wolski, W. (1962). *The Michigan Picture Language Inventory*. Ann Arbor, MI: University of Michigan Press.

Levitt, E. (1957). The results of psychotherapy with children: An evaluation. *Journal of Consulting Psychology, 21*, 189–196.

Levitt, E. (1963). Psychotherapy with children: A further evaluation. *Behaviour Research and Therapy, 1*, 45–51.

Liff, S. (1973). *Early intervention and language development in hearing impaired children*. Unpublished master's thesis, Vanderbilt University.

Liles, B., Shulman, M., & Bartlett, S. (1977). Judgements of grammaticality by normal and language disordered children. *Journal of Speech and Hearing Disorders, 42*, 199–209.

Lillywhite, H., & Bradley, D. (1969). *Communication problems in mental retardation*. New York: Harper & Row.

Lindamood, C. H., & Lindamood, P. C. (1971). *Lindamood Auditory Conceptualization Test*. Boston: Teaching Resources.

Lloyd, L., & Dahle, A. (1976). Detection and diagnosis of a hearing impairment in the child. *Volta Review, 78*, 12–22.

Lodge, D. N., & Leach, E. A. (1975). Children's acquisition of idioms in the English language. *Journal of Speech and Hearing Research, 18*, 521–529.

Lotter, V. (1967). Epidemiology of autistic conditions in young children: I. Prevalence. *Social Psychology, 1*, 163–173.

Lou, H., Brandt, S., & Bruhn, P. (1977). Aphasia and epilepsy in childhood. *Acta Neurologica Scandinavica, 56*, 46–54.

Lovell, K., & Bradbury, B. (1967). The learning of English morphology in educationally subnormal special school children. *American Journal of Mental Deficiency, 71*, 609–615.

Lowe, A., & Campbell, R. (1965). Temporal discrimination in aphasoid and normal children. *Journal of Speech and Hearing Disorders, 30*, 313–314.

Luria, A. (1961). *The role of speech in the regulation of normal and abnormal behavior*. Oxford: Pergamon Press.

Lyle, J. (1961). A comparison of the language of normal and imbecile children. *Journal of Mental Deficiency Research, 5*, 40–51.

Lynch, J. (1979). Use of a prescreening checklist to supplement speech, language, and hearing screening. *Language, Speech, and Hearing Service in Schools, 10*, 249–258.

Maccario, M., Hefferen, S. J., Keblusek, S. J., & Lipinski, K. A. (1982). Developmental dysphasia and electroencephalographic abnormalities. *Developmental Medicine and Child Neurology, 24*, 141–155.

Mantovani, J., & Landau, W. (1980). Acquired aphasia with convulsive disorder: Course and prognosis. *Neurology, 30*, 524–529.

Mark, H. J., & Hardy, W. G. (1958). Orienting reflex disturbances in central auditory or language handicapped children. *Journal of Speech and Hearing Disorders, 223*, 237–242.

Martin, J. (1980). Syndrome delineation in communication disorders. In L. A. Hersov, M. Berger, & E. A. Nicol (Eds.), *Language and language disorders in childhood* (pp. 77–95). New York: Pergamon Press.

Masland, M., & Case, L. (1968). Limitation of auditory memory as a factor in delayed language development. *British Journal of Disorders of Communication, 3*, 139–142.

Matthews, J. (1957). Speech problems of the mentally retarded. In L. Travis (Ed.), *Handbook of speech pathology* (pp. 531–551). New York: Appleton-Century-Crofts.

Mayer, R., & Romanini, M. (1973). Elective mutism. *Neuropsichiatria Infantile, 147*, 717–727.

McDade, H. (1981). A parent–child interactional model for assessing and remediating language disabilities. *British Journal of Disorders of Communication, 16*, 175–183.

McDonald, E. T. (1964). *A Deep Test of Articulation*. Pittsburgh: Stanwyx House.

McDonald, J. D. (1978). *Environmental Language Inventory*. Columbus, OH: Charles E. Merrill.

McGinnis, M. A. (1963). *Aphasic children: Identification and education by the association method*. Washington, DC: Alexander Graham Bell Association for the Deaf.

McGinnis, M. A., Kleffner, F. R., & Goldstein, R. (1956). Teaching aphasic children. *Volta Review, 58*, 239–244.

McGrady, H. (1968). Language pathology and learning disabilities. In H. Myklebust (Ed.), *Progress in learning disabilities* (Vol. 1, pp. 199–233). New York: Grune & Stratton.

McKinney, W., & McGreal, D. (1974). An aphasic syndrome in children. *Canadian Medical Association Journal, 6*, 637–639.

McNeill, D. (1970). *The acquisition of language: The study of developmental psycholinguistics*. New York: Harper & Row.

McReynolds, L. V. (1967). Verbal sequence discrimination training for language impaired children. *Journal of Speech and Hearing Disorders, 32*, 249–256.

McReynolds, L. V. (1978). Behavioral and linguistic considerations in children's speech production. In J. Kavanagh & W. Strange (Eds.), *Speech and language in the laboratory, school, and clinic* (pp. 127–164). Cambridge, MA: M.I.T. Press.

Mecham, M. (1958). *Verbal Language Development Scale*. Minneapolis, MN: Educational Test Bureau.

Mecham, M., Jex, J., & Jones, J. (1967). *Utah Test of Language Development*. Salt Lake City: Communication Research.

Meline, T. J., & Meline, N. C. (1981). Normal variation and prediction of mean length of utterance from chronological age. *Perceptual and Motor Skills, 53*(2), 12–16.

Menyuk, P. (1964). Comparison of grammar of children with functionally deviant and normal speech. *Journal of Speech and Hearing Research, 7*, 109–121.

Menyuk, P. (1971). *The acquisition and development of language*. Englewood Cliffs, NJ: Prentice-Hall.

MIlgram, N. (1966). Verbalization and conceptual classification of trainable mentally retarded children. *American Journal of Mental Deficiency, 70*, 763–765.

Miller, J., Campbell, T., Champa, R., & Weismer, S. (1984). Language behavior in acquired childhood aphasia. In A. Holland (Ed.), *Language disorders in children* (pp. 57–100). San Diego, CA: College Hill.

Mittler, P. (1972). Psychological assessment of language abilities. In M. Rutter & J. Martin (Eds.), *The child with delayed speech* (pp. 106–119). London, England: Spastics International Medical Publications/Heinemann.

Monsees, E. K. (1961). Aphasia in children. *Journal of Speech and Hearing Disorders, 26*, 83–86.

Monsees, E. K. (1968). Temporal sequence and expressive language disorders. *Exceptional Child, 35*, 141–147.

Morehead, D. M., & Ingram, D. (1973). The development of base syntax in normal and linguistically deviant children. *Journal of Speech and Hearing Research, 16*, 330–352.

Morley, M. E. (1957). *The development and disorders of speech in childhood.* Edinburgh: E. & S. Livingstone.

Morley, M. E. (1965). *The development and disorders of speech in childhood* (2nd ed.). Edinburgh: E. & S. Livingstone.

Morton-Evans, A., & Hensley, R. (1978). Paired associate learning in early infantile autism and developmental aphasia. *Journal of Autism and Childhood Schizophrenia, 8,* 61–69.

Mowrer, O. H. (1960). *Learning theory and symbolic processes.* New York: Wiley.

Muller, E., Hollien, H., & Murray, T. (1974). Perceptual responses to infant crying: Identification of cry types. *Journal of Child Language, 1,* 89–95.

Muma, J., & Pierce, S. (1981). Language intervention: Data or evidence. *Topics in Language and Learning Disabilities, 1,* 1–11.

Myklebust, H. R. (1954). *Auditory disorders in children.* New York: Grune & Stratton.

Myklebust, H. R. (1965). *Development and disorders of written language: Vol. 1. Picture Story Language Test.* New York: Grune & Stratton.

Myklebust, H. (1983). Disorders of auditory language. In H. Myklebust (Ed.), *Progress in learning disabilities* (Vol. 5, pp. 45–77). New York: Grune & Stratton.

Nakazima, S. (1975). Phonemicization and symbolization in language development. In E. H. Lenneberg & E. Lenneberg (Eds.), *Foundations of language: A multidisciplinary approach* (Vol. 1, pp. 181–189). New York: Academic Press.

Naremore, R., & Dever, R. (1975). Language performance of educable mentally retarded and normal children at five age levels. *Journal of Speech and Hearing Research, 18,* 82–95.

Nelson, K. (1973). Structure and strategy in learning to talk. *Monographs of the Society for Research in Child Development, 38*(Serial No. 149).

Nelson, K. (1981). Individual differences in language development: Implications for development and language. *Developmental Psychology, 17,* 170–187.

Nelson, K., & Bonvillian, J. (1978). Early language development: Conceptual growth and related processes between 2 and 4½ years of age. In K. Nelson (Ed.), *Children's language* (Vol. 1, pp. 467–556). New York: Gardner Press.

Newcomer, P. L., & Hammill, D. D. (1977). *Test of Language Development (Told).* Austin, TX: Empiric Press.

Northern, J., & Downs, M. (1978). *Hearing in children* (2nd ed.). Baltimore: Williams & Wilkins.

Odom, R. D., Liebert, R. M., & Hill, J. H. (1968). The effects of modelling cues, reward, and attentional set on the production of grammatical and ungrammatical syntactic constructions. *Journal of Experimental Child Psychology, 6,* 131–140.

Oelschlaeger, M., & Scarborough, J. (1976). Traumatic aphasia in children: A case study. *Journal of Communication Disorders, 9,* 281–288.

Oller, D., & Kelly, C. (1974). Phonological substitution processes of a hard of hearing child. *Journal of Speech and Hearing Disorders, 39,* 65–74.

Oller, D. K., Wieman, L. A., Doyle, W. J., & Ross, C. (1976). Infant babbling and speech. *Journal of Child Language, 3,* 1–11.

Orton, S. T. (1937). *Reading, writing and spelling problems in children.* New York: Norton.

Ortony, A., Reynolds, R., & Arter, J. (1978). Metaphor: Theoretical and empirical research. *Psychological Bulletin, 85,* 919–943.

Oviatt, S. (1980). The emerging ability to comprehend language: An experimental approach. *Child Development, 51,* 97–106.

Palermo, D. S., & Molfese, D. L. (1972). Language acquisition from age five onward. *Psychological Bulletin, 68,* 409–428.

Panagos, J. M., & Griffith, P. L. (1981). Okay, what do educators know about language intervention? *Topics in Language and Learning Disabilities, 1*, 69–82.

Patterson, G. (1971). *Families*. Champaign, IL: Research Press.

Patterson, G., & Gullion, M. (1971). *Living with children*. Champaign, IL: Research Press.

Paul, R., Cohen, D. J., & Caparulo, B. K. (1983). A longitudinal study of patients with severe developmental disorders of language learning. *Journal of the American Academy of Child Psychiatry, 22*, 525–534.

Pelham, W. E., Bender, M. E., Caddell, J., & Booth, S. (1984). *The dose response effects of methylphenidate on classroom, academic, and social behavior in hyperactive children*. Unpublished manuscript, Florida State University, Tallahassee.

Pendergast, K., Dickey, S. E., Selmar, J. W., & Soder, A. L. (1969). *Photo Articulation Test*. Danville, IL: Interstate Printers.

Perkins, W. H. (1977). *Speech pathology: An applied behavioral science*. St. Louis: C. V. Mosby.

Petrie, I. (1975). Characteristics and progress of a group of language disordered children with severe receptive difficulties. *British Journal of Disorders of Communication, 10*, 123–133.

Piaget, J. (1926). *Language and thought of the child*. New York: Harcourt, Brace.

Piaget, J. (1952). *The child's conception of number*. London: Routledge & Kegan Paul.

Pirozzolo, F. J., Campanella, D. J., Christensen, K., & Lawson-Kerr, K. (1981). Effects of cerebral dysfunction on neurolinguistic performance in children. *Journal of Consulting and Clinical Psychology, 49*, 791–806.

Pollack, E., & Rees, N. (1972). Disorders of articulation: Some clinical applications of distinctive features. *Journal of Speech and Hearing Disorders, 37*, 451–461.

Poole, I. (1934). Genetic development in articulation of consonant sounds in speech. *Elementary English, 11*, 159–161.

Porch, B. E. (1975). *Porch Index of Communicative Ability in Children (PICAC)*. Palo Alto, CA: Consulting Psychologists Press.

Prather, E. M., Breecher, S., Stafford, M. L., & Wallace, E. M. (1980). *Screening Test of Adolescent Language (STAL)*. Seattle: University of Washington Press.

Prizant, B., & Duchan, J. (1981). The functions of immediate echolalia in autistic children. *Journal of Speech and Hearing Disorders, 46*, 241–249.

Pronovost, W. (1953). *The Boston University Speech Sound Discrimination Test*. Cedar Falls, IA: Go-Mo Products.

Pronovost, W., Wakstein, M., & Wakstein, D. (1966). A longitudinal study of the speech behavior and language comprehension of 14 children diagnosed atypical and autistic. *Exceptional Children, 33*, 19–26.

Puig-Antich, J. (1985). *Kiddie-SADS*. Unpublished manuscript, Western Psychiatric Institute and Clinic, Pittsburgh.

Pustrom, E., & Speers, R. (1964). Elective mutism in children. *Journal of the American Academy of Child Psychiatry, 3*, 287–297.

Quigley, S., Wilbur, R., Power, D., Mantanelli, D., & Steinkamp, M. (1976). *Syntactic structures in the language of deaf children* (Final Report, Project No. 232175). Urbana: University of Illinois.

Rachman, S. (1971). *The effects of psychotherapy*. Oxford: Pergamon Press.

Radloff, L. (1985). *DISC: Diagnostic Interview Schedule for Children*. (Available from Lenore Radloff, Division of Biometry and Epidemiology, Parklawn Building, 5600 Fishers Lane, Bethesda, MD.)

Reagan, C. L., & Cunningham, S. A. (1976). *Differentiation of Auditory Perception Skills (DAPS)*. Tucson, AZ: Communication.

Reed, G. (1963). Elective mutism in children: A reappraisal. *Journal of Child Psychology and Psychiatry and Allied Disciplines, 4,* 99–107.

Reichman, J., & Healey, W. (1983). Learning disabilities and conductive hearing loss involving otitis media. *Journal of Learning Disabilities, 16,* 272–278.

Reynell, J. (1977). *Manual for the Reynell developmental language scales* (rev. ed.). Windsor, England: National Foundation for Educational Research.

Reynell, J. (1979). Pre-language. *Child: Care, Health and Development, 5*(1), 75–80.

Richman, L., & Lindgren, S. (1980). Patterns of intellectual ability in children with verbal deficits. *Journal of Abnormal Child Psychology, 8,* 65–81.

Ricks, D. M. (1975). Vocal communication in preverbal, normal, and autistic children. In N. O'Connor (Ed.), *Language, cognitive deficits, and retardation* (pp. 75–80). London: Butterworths.

Ricks, D. M., & Wing, L. (1976). Language communication and the use of symbols in normal and autistic children. In L. Wing (Ed.), *Early childhood autism* (pp. 93–134). Oxford: Pergamon Press.

Riley, G. D. (1971). *The Riley Articulation and Language Test* (*RALT*). Los Angeles: Western Psychological Services.

Rimland, B. (1978, August). Inside the mind of the autistic savant. *Psychology Today, 12*(3), pp. 69–70, 73–74, 77, 79–80.

Rodda, M. (1977). Language and language disordered children. *Bulletin of British Psychology and Sociology, 30,* 139–142.

Rodgers, W. C. (1976). *Picture Articulation and Language Screening Test.* Salt Lake City, UT: Ward Making Products.

Rogers, M. (1975). A study of language skills in severely subnormal children. *Child: Care, Health and Development, 1,* 113–126.

Rohr, A., & Burr, D. (1978). Etiological differences in patterns of psycholinguistic development of children of IQ 30 to 60. *Journal of Mental Deficiency, 82,* 549–553.

Rondal, J. (1980). The interactive point of view in language development disorders and intervention. *Psychologia Belgica, 20,* 185–204.

Rosenthal, W. S. (1972). Auditory and linguistic interaction in developmental aphasia: Evidence from two studies of auditory processing. *Papers and Reports on Child Language, 4,* 19–34.

Rosner, J. (1979). Screening for perceptual skills dysfunction: An update. *Journal of the American Optometric Association, 50,* 1115–1119.

Ross, D. M., & Ross, S. A. (1982). *Hyperactivity: Current issues, research, and theory.* New York: Wiley.

Roswell, F. G., & Chall, J. S. (1963). *Roswell-Chall Auditory Blending Test.* New York: Essay Press.

Rutter, M. (1966). *Children of sick parents: An environmental and psychiatric study* (Maudsley Monograph No. 16). London: Oxford University Press.

Rutter, M. (1967). Psychotic disorders in early childhood. In A. Coppen & A. Walk (Eds.), *Recent developments in schizophrenia: A symposium* (pp. 133–158). London: Royal Medico-Psychological Association.

Rutter, M. (1978). Language disorder and infantile autism. In M. Rutter & E. Schopler (Eds.), *Autism: Reappraisal of concepts and treatments* (pp. 85–104). New York: Plenum.

Rutter, M., Tuma, H., & Lann, I. (Eds.) (in press). *Assessment, Diagnosis, & Classification in Child & Adolescent Psychopathology.* New York: Guilford Press.

Ryan, J. (1975). Mental subnormality and language development. In E. Lenneberg & E. Lenneberg (Eds.), *Foundations of language and development* (Vol. 2, pp. 269–277). New York: Academic Press.

Salfield, S. (1950). Observations of elective mutism in children. *Journal of Mental Science, 96*, 1024–1032.

Salzinger, S., Patenaude, J., & Lichtenstein, A. (1975). Descriptive study of the effects of selected variables on the communicative speech of pre-school children. *Annals of the New York Academy of Sciences, 263*, 114–131.

Sander, E. K. (1972). When are speech sounds learned? *Journal of Speech and Hearing Disorders, 37*, 55–63.

Sato, S., & Dreifuss, F. E. (1973). Electroencephalographic findings in a patient with developmental expressive aphasia. *Neurology, 23*, 181–185.

Satz, P., & Morris, R. (1981). LD subtypes: A review. In F. Pirozzolo & N. Wittrock (Eds.), *Neuropsychological and cognitive processes in reading* (pp. 109–141). New York: Academic Press.

Savage, V. (1968). Childhood autism: A review of the literature with particular reference to the speech and language structure of the autistic child. *British Journal of Disorders of Communication, 3*, 75–87.

Schere, R. A., Richardson, E., & Bialer, I. (1980). Toward operationalizing a psychoeducational definition of LD. *Journal of Abnormal Child Psychology, 8*, 5–20.

Schiefelbusch, R. (1972). Language disabilities of cognitively involved children. In J. Irwin & M. Marge (Eds.), *Principles of childhood language disabilities* (pp. 209–237). Englewood Cliffs, NJ: Prentice-Hall.

Schlesinger, H., & Meadow, K. (1972). *Sound and sign: Childhood deafness and mental health.* Berkeley: University of California Press.

Schneider, K. (1959). *Critical psychopathology*. New York: Grune & Stratton.

Schuler, A. (1980). Aspects of communication. In W. Fay & A. Schuler (Eds.), *Emerging language in autistic children* (pp. 89–111). Baltimore: University Park Press.

Schwartz, A. H., & Murphy, M. W. (1975). Cues for screening language disorders in preschool children. *Pediatrics, 55*, 717–722.

Schwartz, R., Leonard, L., Folger, M., & Wilcox, M. (1980). Early phonological behavior in normal-speaking and language disordered children: Evidence for a synergistic view of linguistic disorders. *Journal of Speech and Hearing Disorders, 45*, 357–377.

Schwartz, S. (1982). Is there a schizophrenic language? *Behavioral and Brain Sciences, 5*, 579–626.

Semel, E. (1976). *Semel Auditory Processing Program*. Chicago: Follett.

Semel, E., & Wiig, E. (1980a). *CELF: Clinical Evaluation of Language Functions: Diagnostic Battery*. Columbus, OH: Charles E. Merrill.

Semel, E., & Wiig, E. (1980b). *CELF: Clinical Evaluation of Language Functions: Screening Test*. Columbus, OH: Charles E. Merrill.

Semel, E., & Wiig, E. (1981). Semel Auditory Processing Program: Training effects among children with language-learning disabilities. *Journal of Learning Disabilities, 14*, 192–196.

Semmel, M. I., Barritt, L. S., & Bennett, S. W. (1970). Performance of EMR and nonretarded children on modified close task. *American Journal of Mental Deficiency, 74*, 681–688.

Semmel, M. I., & Dolley, D. G. (1971). Comprehension and imitation of sentences by Downs syndrome children as a function of transformational complexity. *American Journal of Mental Deficiency, 75*, 739–745.

Shaffer, D., & Greenhill, L. (1979). A critical note on the predictive validity of the hyperkinetic syndrome. *Journal of Child Psychology, 20*, 61–72.

Shapiro, T., Roberts, A., & Fish, B. (1970). Imitation and echoing in young schizophrenic children. *Journal of the American Academy of Child Psychiatry, 9*, 548–567.

Shelton, R. (1978). The use of research in the development of clinical services for individuals with speech disorders. In J. Kavanagh & W. Strange (Eds.), *Speech and language in the laboratory, school, and clinic* (pp. 165–178). Cambridge, MA: MIT Press.

Shelton, R., Arndt, W., & Miller, J. (1961). Learning principles and the teaching of speech and language. *Journal of Speech and Hearing Disorders, 26*, 368–376.

Sheridan, M., & Peckham, C. (1975). Follow-up at 11 years of children who had marked speech defects at 7 years. *Child: Care, Health and Development, 113*, 157–166.

Sheridan, M., & Peckham, C. (1978). Follow-up to 16 years of school children who had marked speech defects at 7 years. *Child: Care, Health and Development, 4*, 145–157.

Shervanian, C. (1967). Speech, thought, and communication disorders in childhood psychosis: Theoretical implications. *Journal of Speech and Hearing Disorders, 32*, 303–313.

Shoumaker, R., Bennett, D., Bray, D., & Curless, G. (1974). Clinical and EEG manifestations of an unusual aphasic syndrome in children. *Neurology, 24*, 10–16.

Silverman, S. (1971). The education of deaf children. In L. Travis (Ed.), *Handbook of speech pathology and audiology* (pp. 399–430). New York: Appleton-Century-Crofts.

Simmons, A. (1962). Comparison of the type-token ratio of spoken and written language of deaf and hearing children. *Volta Review, 64*, 417–421.

Simmons, J., & Tymchuk, A. (1973). The learning deficits in childhood psychosis. *Pediatric Clinics of North America, 20*, 665–679.

Simon, N. (1975). Echolalic speech in childhood autism. *Archives of General Psychiatry, 32*, 1439–1446.

Snow, K. (1963). A detailed analysis of articulation responses of "normal" first grade children. *Journal of Speech and Hearing Research, 6*, 277–290.

Sowell, V., Parker, R., Poplin, M., & Larsen, S. (1979). The effects of psycholinguistic training on improving psycholinguistic skills. *Learning Disability Quarterly, 2*(3), 69–77.

Spencer, E. M. (1958). *An investigation of the maturation of various factors of auditory perception in pre-school children*. Unpublished doctoral dissertation, Northwestern University.

Spradlin, J. (1963). Assessment of speech language of retarded children: The Parsons language sample. *Journal of Speech and Hearing Disorders Monographs, 10*, 8–31.

Spradlin, J., & McLean, J. (1967). *Linguistics and retardation*. Unpublished manuscript, Bureau of Child Research, Parson, KS.

Spradlin, J., & Siegel, G. (1982). Language training in natural and clinical environments. *Journal of Speech and Hearing Disorders, 47*, 2–6.

Spreen, O. (1965). Language functions in mental retardation: A review. *American Journal of Mental Deficiency, 69*, 482–494.

Stark, J., Poppen, R., & May, M. Z. (1967). Effects of alterations of prosodic features on the sequencing performance of aphasic children. *Journal of Speech and Hearing Research, 10*, 849–855.

Stern, D. N., Jaffe, J., Beebe, B., & Bennett, S. L. (1975). Vocalizing in unison and in alternation: Two modes of communication within the mother–infant dyad. *Annals of the New York Academy of Sciences, 263*, 89–100.

Stevenson, J., & Richman, N. (1976). The prevalence of language delay in a population of three-year old children and its association with general retardation. *Developmental Medicine and Child Neurology, 18*, 431–441.

Stevenson, J., Richman, N., & Graham, P. (1985). Behaviour problems and language abilities at three years and behavioural deviance at eight years. *Journal of Child Psychology and Psychiatry and Allied Disciplines, 26*, 215–230.

Stewart, M., & Olds, S. (1973). *Raising a hyperactive child*. New York: Harper & Row.

Strauss, A. A. (1954). Aphasia in children. *American Journal of Physical Medicine, 33*, 93–99.

Tallal, P. (1978). Implications of speech perceptual research for clinical population: A discussion of Cutting and Pisoni's paper. In J. Kavanagh & W. Strange (Eds.), *Speech and language in the laboratory, school, and clinic* (pp. 73–88). Cambridge, MA: M.I.T. Press.

Templin, M. C. (1956). Sound discrimination test. In M. F. Berry & J. Eisenson, *Speech Disorders* (Appendix 3). New York: Appleton-Century-Crofts.

Templin, M. C. (1957). *Certain language skills in children* (Institute of Child Welfare Monograph Serial No. 26). Minneapolis: University of Minnesota Press.

Templin, M., & Darley, F. (1969). *The Templin–Darley Tests of Articulation*. Iowa City: Bureau of Educational Research and Services, University of Iowa.

Thorum, A. R. (1980). *The Fullerton Language Test for Adolescents*. Palo Alto, CA: Consulting Psychologists Press.

Todd, G., & Palmer, B. (1968). Social reinforcement of infant babbling. *Child Development, 39*, 591–595.

Tomblin, J. B. (1978). Children's language disorders. In J. Curtis (Ed.), *Processes and disorders of human communication* (pp. 246–271). New York: Harper & Row.

Toronto, A. S. (1977a). *Southwestern Spanish Articulation Test*. Austin, TX: Academy Tests.

Toronto, A. S. (1977b). *Toronto Tests of Receptive Vocabulary: English/Spanish* (*TTRV*). Austin, TX: Academy Tests.

Toronto, A. S., Leverman, D., Hanna, C., Rosenzweig, P., & Maldonado, A. (1975). *Del Rio Language Screening Test English/Spanish*. Austin, TX: National Education Laboratory.

Tramer, M. (1934). Elektiver mutismusbei kindern. *Zeitschrift für Kinderpsychiatrie, 1*, 30–35.

Trantham, C. R., & Pedersen, J. K. (1976). *Normal language development: The key to diagnosis and therapy for language disordered children*. Baltimore: Williams & Wilkins.

Tubbs, V. (1966). Types of linguistic disability in psychotic children. *Journal of Mental Deficiency Research, 10*, 230–240.

U. S. Public Law 94-142 (The Education of the Handicapped Act). (1975).

Vaisse, L. (1866). Des lourds-muets de certains cas d'aphasie congénitale. *Bulletin de la Société d'Anthropologie de Paris, 1*, 146–150.

VanDongen, H., & Loonen, M. (1977). Factors related to prognosis of acquired aphasia in children. *Cortex, 13*, 131–136.

Van Kleeck, A. (1984). Metalinguistic skills: Cutting across spoken and written language and problem-solving abilities. In G. Wallach & K. Butler (Eds.), *Language learning disabilities in school-age children* (pp. 128–153). Baltimore: Williams & Wilkins.

Wallach, G. P. (1984). Later language learning: Syntactic structures and strategies. In G. Wallach & K. Butler (Eds.), *Language learning disabilities in school-age children* (pp. 82–102). Baltimore: Williams & Wilkins.

Wanderley, E., & Lefevre, A. (1969). Aphasia acquired in childhood. *Arquivos de Neuro-Psiquiatria, 27*, 87–96.

Watters, G. (1974). The syndrome of acquired aphasia and convulsive disorder in children. *Canadian Medical Journal, 16*, 110–111.

Wechsler, D. (1967). *Wechsler Pre-school and Primary Scale of Intelligence* (*WPPSI*). New York: Psychological Corporation.

Wechsler, D. (1974). *Wechsler Intelligence Scale for Children—Revised* (*WISC*-R). New York: Psychological Corporation.

Weiner, F. (1981). Systematic sound preference as a characteristic of phonological disability. *Journal of Speech and Hearing Disorders, 46*, 281–286.

Weiss, C., & Lillywhite, H. (1981). *Communicative disorders: Prevention and early intervention*. St. Louis: C. V. Mosby.

Welner, Z. (1985). *DICA: Diagnostic Interview for Children and Adolescents*. Unpublished

manuscript, Washington University School of Medicine, Division of Child Psychiatry.
Wender, P., & Wender, E. (1978). *The hyperactive and learning disabled child.* New York: Crown Press.
Wepman, J. (1973). *Auditory Discrimination Test.* Chicago: Language Research Associates.
Wepman, J., & Morency, A. (1975). *The Auditory Sequential Memory Test.* Chicago: Language Research Associates.
Wergeland, H. (1979). Elective mutism. *Acta Psychiatrica Scandinavica, 59,* 218–228.
Werry, J. (1979). The childhood psychoses. In H. Quay & J. Werry (Eds.), *Psychopathologic disorders of childhood* (pp. 43–89). New York: Wiley.
West, J., & Weber, J. (1974). A linguistic analysis of the morphemic and syntactic structure of a hard of hearing child. *Language and Speech, 17,* 68–79.
Wiig, E., & Semel, E. (1973). Comprehension of linguistic concepts requiring logical operations by learning disabled children. *Journal of Speech and Hearing Research, 16,* 627–636.
Wiig, E., & Semel, E. (1976). *Language disabilities in children and adolescents.* Columbus, OH: Charles E. Merrill.
Wiig, E., & Semel, E. (1980). *Language assessment and intervention for the learning disabled.* Columbus, OH: Carles E. Merrill.
Wilson, J., Rapin, J., Wilson, B., & VanDenburg, F. (1975). Neuropsychologic function of children with severe hearing impairment. *Journal of Speech and Hearing Research, 18,* 634–651.
Wing, L. (1969). The handicaps of autistic children: A comparative study. *Journal of Child Psychology and Psychiatry and Allied Disciplines, 10,* 1–40.
Winitz, H. (1969). *Articulatory acquisition and behavior.* Englewood Cliffs, NJ: Prentice-Hall.
Witelson, S., & Rabinovitz, M. S. (1972). Hemispheric speech lateralization in children with auditory linguistic deficits. *Cortex, 8,* 412–426.
Wolff, S., & Chess, S. (1965). An analysis of the language of 14 schizophrenic children. *Journal of Child Psychology and Psychiatry and Allied Disciplines, 6,* 29–41.
Wolfus, B., Moscovitch, M., & Kinsbourne, M. (1980). Subgroups of developmental language impairment. *Brain and Language, 10,* 152–171.
Wolpaw, T., Nation, J., & Aram, D. (1979). Developmental language disorders: A follow-up study. *Illinois Speech and Hearing Journal, 12,* 14–18.
Wood, N. E. (1964). *Delayed speech and language development.* Englewood Cliffs, NJ: Prentice Hall.
Woods, B., & Carey, S. (1979). Language deficits after apparent clinical recovery from childhood aphasia. *Annals of Neurology, 6,* 405–409.
World Health Organization. (1977). *International classification of diseases* (9th ed.). Geneva: Author.
Worster-Drought, C. (1971). An unusual form of acquired aphasia in children. *Developmental Medicine and Child Neurology, 13,* 563–571.
Wright, H. (1968). A clinical study of children who refuse to talk in school. *Journal of the American Academy of Child Psychiatry, 7,* 603–617.
Yeni-Komshian, G. (1977). A longterm study of dichotic speech perception and receptive language skills in a child with acquired aphasia. In S. Segalowitz & F. Gruber (Eds.), *Language development and neurological theory* (pp. 145–154). New York: Academic Press.
Yoder, D., & Miller, J. (1972). What we may know and what we can do: Input toward a system. In J. McLean, D. Yoder, & R. Schiefelbusch (Eds.), *Language intervention with the retarded* (pp. 89–107). Baltimore: University Park Press.
Yule, W., & Berger, M. (1972). Behavior modification principles and speech delay. In

M. Rutter & J. Martin (Eds.), *The child with delayed speech* (pp. 204–219). London: Spastics International Medical Publications/Heinemann.

Zachman, L., Huisingh, R., Jorgensen, C., & Barrett, M. (1977). *The Oral Language Sentence Imitation Test (OLSIT) and the Oral Language Sentence Imitation Diagnostic Inventory (OLSDI)*. Moline, IL: Linguistic Systems.

Zaidel, E. (1979). The split and half brains as models of congenital language disability. In C. L. Ludlow & M. E. Doran-Quine (Eds.), *The neurological bases of language disorders in children: Methods and directions for research* (pp. 55–90). Washington, DC: U. S. Department of Health, Education, and Welfare.

Zigmond, N., Vallecorsa, A., & Leinhardt, G. (1982). Reading instruction for students with learning disabilities. In K. Butler & G. Wallach (Eds.), *Language disorders and learning disabilities* (pp. 89–98). Baltimore: Aspen.

Zimmerman, I. L., Steiner, V. G., & Evatt, R. (1969). *Preschool Language Scale*. Columbus, OH: Charles E. Merrill.

INDEX